Sick In Shadows

CATHY ANN ROGERS

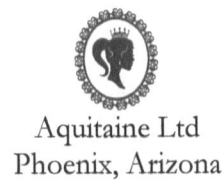

Aquitaine Ltd
Phoenix, Arizona

This is a work of fiction. Names, characters, businesses, places, events and incidents are either the products of the author's imagination or used in a fictitious manner. Any resemblance to actual persons, living or dead, or actual events is purely coincidental.

Sally J Smith, Editor
Cover design by JD Smith Designs

Copyright © 2015 Cathy Ann Rogers

ISBN-10: 0-9914843-8-X
ISBN-13: 978-09914843-8-6

www.aquitaineltd.com

DEDICATION

For the *real* Lord of Plastic Surgery

"She made three paces through the room,
She saw the water-lily bloom,
She saw the helmet and the plume,
She looked down to Camelot.
Out flew the web and floated wide;
The mirror cracked from side to side;
"The curse is come upon me," cried
The Lady of Shalott."

LORD ALFRED TENNYSON

The Lady of Shalott

Delia Ferguson took Polly's delicate hands in her own and squeezed. The woman who sat opposite Delia at the small office table looked up at her with a weak smile. Delia released her grasp, closed her eyes, and placed her palms on the wooden surface.

"Delia, what do you see?"

Not since she had assumed the title of intuitive therapist to complement her conventional practice in social work had she been afraid. She often encountered Polly's type of fretful unhappiness in other clients, sensing a dark hollow in them that stemmed from a life lived in fear or insecurity. Employing her empathetic talents, Delia embraced their burdens to draw out the source of their suffering and guide them into a brighter emotional space. She accepted that plunging into their darkness had risks, but she had never let that worry her until she met Polly.

Clients did not always come to her to clear what blocked them from being happy. On occasion, they demanded support and validation for the dangerous path they had chosen or were about to choose. Delia took pride in leading them away from their sinister nature. But Polly paralyzed her, had a stronger will. Delia shivered, but she knew what she must do. Another person's safety depended on her. She had to tell the police.

"Polly, I think you need to consider the consequences. Harming others to protect him, well, that's not a foundation for a strong relationship."

"Are you going to tell?"

Delia met the other woman's eyes and smiled, but she could not control the quiver of her lip. "Of course not. What we talk about is confidential. Besides, I have no way to know if you intend to do any of this or if you're working out your frustrations by creating fantasies. Fantasizing is not a crime."

"You're not the only intuitive in this room, Delia. You're going to call the police as soon as you hear about it on the news. Maybe you'll call once I leave this room. I can't have that."

"What are you suggesting? That you would harm me? You would go that far to keep your secret?"

"I'm not *suggesting* anything."

Delia looked into Polly's eyes. The evil she saw there ripped through her. She had to get out now.

Delia rose to make a dash to the door. Polly blocked her way. As if they had the same thought, both heads turned toward the shelf by the door. Polly grabbed the crystal skull first. Delia watched Polly's arm swing toward her. She froze, terrified. Then the bone shattering sound when the glass orb made contact with her head. Disoriented, arms flailing, knees folding under her, Delia started the descent to the floor.

CHAPTER ONE

Imogen Vine stared down at her new breasts and then across to her nude reflection in the full-length mirror. She moved her hands over her new nipples, down her sides and over her tummy, turning to the side for a better look. The transformation continued to fascinate her after the destruction she experienced from cancer in her right breast. She had opted to have both breasts removed after her cousin had developed breast cancer in her second breast seventeen years after the first diagnosis. The decision had been the right one—she knew that. But the surgery meant to extend her life had also taken her femininity.

She had mourned the loss of the shapeliness that she counted on and took for granted all her life. She had not been able to get past that butchered feeling when she saw her nude body in the mirror. She wanted to be above vanity, but the gnawing sorrow went beyond the simple concern for her looks—it had come down to her sense of identity, as if she were no longer a real woman.

She wiped a tear to protect the heavy eye makeup she had applied for the event. She pulled her silver V-neck dress up over her thighs and hooked it in place. Glimmering beads on silk, a plunging neckline and empire waist to an above-the-knee hemline—she admired her figure from every angle before giving her make-up one last touchup and slipping into her heels.

She reached for a small pad covered with notes and began to put the procedure name to memory in anticipation of the speech she would give at the fundraiser. Her plastic surgeon and close family friend, Tate Marsdon, had created her beautiful new body using an innovative technique with liposuction that used her own body fat to reform her breasts without implants. A post-procedure flap reconstruction provided the added benefit of a taut stomach, as if she had a tummy tuck. New breasts, slimmer belly—modern medicine gave her back the body nature had given her. Before Henry, before the children, before cancer and gravity became her enemy.

She stared at her figure, reflecting at how we define ourselves by our physical appearance, even while we protest that our inner qualities are what matter most. How many times had she preached to her children to stop worrying about their looks and to concentrate on their schoolwork? But she had also raised them to embrace Christian generosity and a gracious attitude toward others. They could have thrown her words back at her, but instead, they had been her biggest supporters, encouraging her to have the reconstruction. Maybe they saw the truth that pride of appearance is not always about vanity.

"Oh, *la joie de vivre.*" She winked at her reflection. She viewed the future with a renewed joy for living. Then she saw her husband, Henry, out of the corner of her eye, stretched across the bed. She frowned and added a mental note to find the best way to get rid of him. Nothing would ever be the same again. *Just ignore him for now. Pretend he is not there.* She had endless possibilities in front of her. She could not let him ruin things. She had to deal with him sooner or later, but not tonight. When she saw her taxi out front, she took a deep breath before shutting off the lights and closing the front door behind her.

"Imogen," Monica Ames said. "You look marvelous." Monica had known Imogen since high school, and they had remained close friends over the years. "I'd go so far as to say you're ravishing."

"I do what I can, dear." Imogen gave Monica a mischievous wink and reached out for a Chardonnay from the passing tray. "It looks as if we have a great turnout. You never know with the economy."

"Yeah, that's true. Still, I heard we've exceeded last year's takings. So, are you going to tell me where Henry is? Did he decide to stay outside with the new car to make sure no one dings it?"

"Henry won't be coming." Imogen said. "I left him in bed."

Monica recognized the abrupt manner Imogen used to end a subject she wanted to avoid, but she decided to needle her about it anyway.

"Yes, it's difficult for a man to make that choice between his wife and his car. Still, I'm surprised he didn't want to be here for your big speech. A little support would've been nice."

"Forget him. He's history as far as I'm concerned."

"Not again. What happened this time?"

"I don't want to talk about it, so stop questioning me," Imogen said. "Oh, look. There's Elle and Simon. I'm going to pop over and say hello."

Monica stood still as she watched her friend glide between the other guests on her way to the other side of the room. It had been a long time since she had seen Imogen under the sort of stress where she would be rude.

To others maybe, but not to her. That must have been one big fight.

Monica raised her wine glass to her lips and caught sight of Dr. Tate. She gave him a smile and nod of acknowledgment. Those piercing dark eyes and wide smile always gave her a jolt. Dr. Tate Marsden, also known as Dr. Tate by his regular patients over the years, had performed the reconstructive surgery on Imogen, as well as the lesser cosmetic surgery procedures on most of their immediate circle of friends. Monica smiled to herself that she still could not figure if he knew how attractive he was or if he discounted the attention of his female patients as the result of the intimacy that develops between doctor and patient. Monica tended to think it was a bit of both.

Monica tilted her head back to drain the last of her wine and picked up another on her way over to his group. She recognized Judge Barry Bellows and his wife Lorraine, who, Monica remembered, became involved in their charity when the Judge lost a sister to breast cancer. A striking redhead stood next to Tate. Not only did she have beauty but a presence not overshadowed by her prominent company. Monica tried to find a flaw, but gave up. Some women either did not need fixing, or their confidence made them appear flawless.

"Hey, Monica. You look great," Tate said. "You know the Bellows, of course, and this is Erin Fitzgerald."

Monica and Erin shook hands. "Nice to meet you," Monica said. The direct eye contact with Erin's green eyes took her back. She had charisma and a bearing that did not intimidate but instead compelled Monica to want to be her friend. "We're having a great turnout. I hope all of you brought your checkbooks."

Monica found Erin intriguing. She tried to study her

without anyone noticing. A long, slender woman with waist-length auburn hair pulled up into a tight ponytail and allowed to hang sensually down the small of her naked waist exposed by the low open back of her floor-length periwinkle silk dress. Monica liked her despite her proprietary gesture of taking Tate's arm at Monica's approach.

"I'm glad you're here," Tate said. "We were just talking about the work you and Imogen put into this fundraiser."

"It's been a great turnout for the Half Marathon and the after party. We've exceeded last year's totals and our expectations," Monica said. She could not stop sipping her wine and hoped she had time to eat before the alcohol went to her head.

"You've both done a great job," Tate said. "By the way, where's Imogen? I thought I saw you both talking a few minutes ago."

"The last time I saw her, she had gone to speak to Simon and Elle Iverson."

Monica looked around but was not able to see Imogen although the Iversons were near them. "Imogen seems stressed this evening. She's not herself, and Henry didn't come. I think there must have been an argument."

"I hope everything's cleared up before tomorrow," Tate said. "They invited me for dinner."

"I'm going to look for her. Excuse me," Monica said. After bowing out from the group, she went into the Ladies Room. Imogen sat on one of the chairs staring into her compact mirror.

"What's up? Dr. Tate asked about you."

"Nothing's up. I wanted a break, that's all."

"We both need to eat. Let's get a plate of food, find a cozy corner and chat."

Imogen sighed and looked up at Monica. "Okay."

"You're starting to creep me out. What's going on with you?"

"I said *nothing*. Stop questioning me, or I'm not going to talk to you."

"Wow," Monica said. "All right. Let's get some food then." Something told her this evening would hit a few speed bumps before it was over.

On the way to the buffet table, Imogen spotted Dr. Tate and changed course toward him.

"Imogen," Tate said. "I didn't recognize you with your clothes on."

Monica started to laugh. He and Imogen exchanged that kind of lighthearted teasing often, but Imogen looked at him with a confused expression. After several tense seconds, Imogen choked out a laugh, but by that time, Tate and the rest of the group had noticed the awkward hesitation.

Barry Bellows, used to taking conciliatory action, changed the subject. "Tate, I've meant to tell you for a long time how much my wife and I admire the work you've done donating your time to perform free breast reconstructions. You're a credit to your field. Wish we had more plastic surgeons like you."

"Plastic surgeon! In your examining room, you said you were a gynecologist." Imogen stopped to observe her audience. Everyone in close proximity to them turned to look. Their halted conversations created a hushed tension around the room. Imogen started belting out hysterical cackling. Monica saw the red flush on Tate's face, while everyone else stared at Imogen waiting for her to speak again.

Monica heard her own sharp intake of breath and closed her eyes. She heard Erin say to Tate, "You had that coming, sweetie." When Monica opened her eyes at last, she saw her friend still laughing, tears pouring from her eyes.

Tate's jaw still gaped open. Monica gave him and the others a helpless look before taking Imogen's arm and leading her outside to the lobby. She did not know what to do but she was certain she would not ask Imogen any more questions. Monica stood with her until she stopped giggling and went quiet. Imogen did not seem to be present. Monica could not allow her give her speech in this state.

Imogen had an odd vibe about her this evening—an uncharacteristic emotional detachment. Monica used her furious texting skills to inform the event's moderator that Imogen would not be able to give her speech, and then led her friend outside to the passenger seat of her car and drove her home.

When she stopped the car in front of Imogen's house, Monica started to get out, but Imogen protested. "I'm alright. You don't need to come in. Besides, Henry's in bed, and I don't want him disturbed."

"Sure, Imogen. Anything you want. You know that." Monica reached over to hug the other woman. She had a bad feeling she could not shake all the way back to the fundraiser.

Once inside her house, Imogen sighed again. It was right for Monica to bring her home. Her behavior went out of control, and she knew it. That she had not been able to recognize it while it happened worried her. She had a problem, but no matter how much she strained to remember, the farther away the answer drew. She walked through the house turning off lights and checking the doors. She worried that Monica would be angry with her and started to cry. When she got to the bedroom, she left the light off so she did not wake Henry. As she passed the bed on the way to the bathroom, she thought of how disgusting he was. Looking forward to the day he was gone consumed her thoughts.

She washed away the day's make-up and brushed her teeth—part of her nightly routine. This ritual had become so mechanical that she finished before she realized any time passed. Something gnawed at her. A sense that she had a big problem, but she could not place it. Then she noticed a familiar smell coming from the bedroom. Oh, my God, she thought. He really is a disgusting man. She sprayed air freshener in the bathroom and on her way out of the bedroom. She grabbed a blanket from the hallway closet and went to sleep on the sofa in the den. Her last thought before falling asleep was of the checklist of items needed for Dr. Tate's dinner tomorrow.

Tate arrived for dinner at the Vine house at seven. He expected to see Henry open the door as usual, but Imogen appeared instead. "I'm sorry but Henry won't be joining us," she said. "He's not well."

A stench hit his nose when he walked across the threshold—a musty, suffocating odor combined with a chemical deodorizer. He leaned in to hug her and sniffed, unsure how he could enjoy the meal with that hovering smell.

"You had me worried last night."

"I'm sorry about that. I don't know what was wrong with me, to tell the truth. I'm embarrassed. I'm sorry if I embarrassed you."

"Don't worry about me. I'm just glad to see you're

okay."

"I'm great. So, do you want to play cards?"

Her abrupt change confused him. Tate tried to read her face for a hint of amusement or the crack of a smile. Nothing but a fixed stare and impassive expression that chilled him. He sniffed the air again and thought that considering the overwhelming stink of the place, avoiding a sit down meal might be a good idea.

"Sure. What card game?"

"Hearts or Spades. I don't care," Imogen said. Tate watched her eyes lose focus briefly, and then she said, "Now where are those cards? Wait a minute. Where's my head? You came for dinner, not cards. Right?"

"I came to visit," Tate said. The hairs bristled on the back of his neck. Something was not right. He shifted into the clinical observer. Her manner tonight was much like the evening before—confused and disoriented. He needed to get Henry out here.

"You said Henry was ill? I *am* a doctor, you know. I even went to school and learned first aid. Why don't I go check on him to see if there's something I can do to help?"

"No!" she said. "He doesn't need help."

Any doubts he might have had about her being in crisis vanished. He wondered if Henry had moved out. Did they have an argument and he left to cool off? Tate had a concern being here alone with her in this state. Under normal circumstances, he saw her as a witty, charming woman full of life with a comely attractiveness, but secure enough in her own femininity that she would not stoop to desperate measures in a bid for attention by trying to turn their friendship into anything beyond that. But these were not normal circumstances. He wanted someone else to be present. Like a witness.

"It's okay, Imogen. I won't bother him," Tate said. He stalled to give himself time to think of something to do.

Her behavior reminded him of a friend who had post-traumatic stress disorder, or PTSD. His friend had been in the fray in Afghanistan, almost killed by a suicide bomber, and had watched the limbs and other body parts of his friends flung through the smoky blur of gunpowder, gasoline fumes, and dirt. A definable incident.

Imogen, a middle-class housewife, had tense moments following the discovery of the cancer, but she had survived the diagnosis and treatment, followed by the reconstructive surgery. She had stress and shock in the beginning like anyone had facing a potentially life-threatening condition. So why now? What in her life could traumatize her? All he knew was that whatever the cause and effect, she had something psychologically or medically wrong with her.

She sat there watching him—both of them breathing in that disgusting smell. Then, like an alarm exploding in his ear, he thought he knew. In that place hovering between fear and repulsion, he realized that the deodorizer was an attempt to cover the odor of rotting corpse. He prepared to subdue her if necessary, but he had to find the body.

She looked at him, reading his thoughts. "No! I refuse."

"Imogen, where's Henry? I need to know right now."

She gave herself away when she glanced at the bedroom. Tate started to walk in that direction. She jumped up and grabbed his arm to pull him back. Instead of struggling to get away from her, he took her arms and forced her toward the bedroom with him. The closer they got, the more violent her struggles until they reached the bedroom door. She stopped struggling, looked up at him, and dropped her arms. She looked frozen.

Tate inched open the bedroom door slowly and felt for the light switch. That confusing contradiction of commercial deodorizer and decomposition hit his olfactory senses. He knew what he would find before the visual confirmation.

He flipped on the wall switch. He saw the *Navaja* blade, Henry's favorite hunting knife first. Tate remembered how Henry had explained the history of the Andalusian folding knife and had described in detail the extensive damage potential of the clip-point edge. This one had a feminine ivory handle with a five and a half inch blade engraved in an ornate style with a man on a horse and the word *"Bandito"* scrolled across the edge. First impressions were that you were looking at an elegant and fragile work of art, but the truth was its façade disguised its potential destructive capacity.

The blade lay exposed on the bed next to Henry, but his blood covered its engraved design. Red smears on the handle cast a vulgar contrast between the dark crustiness of the dried blood and the purity of the translucent polished ivory. Tate knew Henry was dead, but he had to confirm. He stood by the side of the bed, careful not to touch anything else, and placed his two fingers on Henry's neck. His assumptions proved right—no pulse, no warmth, only the death pallor, the bloating in the abdomen, and the discoloration in the veins.

The sensory shock as well as the emotional impact of what had happened in this room overrode his natural ability to control his emotions. He wanted to give into the irrational desire to run. He took a step back from the bed. He looked behind him, saw the bathroom, and knew he could not hold it together any longer. He rushed inside, raised the toilet lid, and threw up.

Tate straightened himself and backed out of the room. Once in the hall, he pulled out his cell phone and dialed 911. After a brief description of the situation, he shut off the call and looked at Imogen who had moved to the living room where she sat motionless and silent. He had no idea how to approach her, or if he should. He stood still to plan his next actions. Psychology was not his forte, nor did he want it to be. He had a natural talent for remodeling and repairing bodies—an inherent gift for healing that came easily. On the other side, the soft sciences that dealt with emotions, behaviors, and impulses left him unimpressed as a field of subjective and speculative theories without absolute definition.

Without doubt, Tate knew he was out of his element, so he chose to do what made the most sense to him. Imogen needed to stay out of that bedroom and to remain calm until the police arrived. He walked down the hall, sat across from her on the settee, and said, "Imogen, are you all right?"

She seemed to react to the sound of his voice, but did not show a comprehension of what he had said. She spoke softly, her eyes distant and unfocussed. "Pretty boy. So kind," she said, and exhaled a deep sigh.

He flinched at her uncharacteristic personal remark, "I try to be kind to my friends."

In what turned out to be a moment of clarity, Imogen started speaking in her soft, even-toned voice. "We were having an argument about something, maybe money. I think I blacked out. I remember feeling tired. I saw his *Navaja* knife open on the dresser. It called out to me. I picked it up and stabbed him in the chest. When he staggered backward, I stabbed him a couple more times to be sure."

Tate had an urge to strike her to make her stop reciting the gruesome details.

"He finally stopped talking," she said. "He put his hand over the bleeding and fell back on the bed. When he looked at me, I told him it served him right for talking to me that way. It *was* the only way to stop him."

After the interviews with police, Tate drove home, exhausted, angry, mournful, but most of all confused. Watching Imogen disappear behind a veil of bewilderment had leveled him. Her ability to reason gone, replaced with a basic survival instinct. He had lost a good friend in Henry Vine, but to realize at the same time that Henry and Imogen might not be the people he thought he knew and that something hidden in the blur of shadows provoked his death, gave his grief an acute bitterness. He poured a large Chivas Scotch, sank into his brown leather chair, and stared out at the city lights beyond his balcony.

He watched the flickering traffic signals moving north and south on Scottsdale Road, and took a few more sips before gulping down the rest of the golden liquid. He set the tumbler on the table next to him and noticed his hands trembling. Unlike his typical controlled demeanor, his emotions had taken on a life of their own. Nervous and anxious, he had no idea how to calm down.

He saw his cell phone light come on indicating an incoming call. He knew he could not face a conversation with anyone right now. Instead of answering, he walked past Erin's photo flashing on the screen, and poured himself another drink. When he sat down again, he reached for his phone and texted Erin, "Imogen murdered Henry. I found his body. Can't talk right now."

CHAPTER TWO

Tate drove through traffic numb and dazed on his way to the office the next morning. He suffered body blows all night from the horrific bedroom scene that spooled in front of him in the darkness as he lay in bed, Henry's body more distorted and amplified as the night passed into morning.

"Good morning, Dr. Marsdon," Rachelle said. Her perky demeanor and soothing attractiveness as their office manager and front office receptionist served as a beacon for his patients that he appreciated. Today, though, her cheerfulness annoyed him. He did his best to disguise irritation that had nothing to do with her and everything to do with him. Not ready to talk about what happened, he forced out the routine salutation through his dry throat.

"Good morning, Rachelle. Do I have any messages?"

"Erin left a message late yesterday, but nothing this morning that I can't handle. I put her message on your desk. Can I get you coffee or something? You look a little rough, like you're coming down with something."

He stiffened at the transparency of his fatigue and emotional strain. He forced a smile. The wall clock read eight forty-five. "No, I'm fine. What's my schedule today?"

"You have appointments until noon. Then you're

open the rest of the day."

"Thanks. I'll be in my office. Let me know when my first patient arrives."

"Sure, doctor."

He felt her eyes follow him down the corridor.

He paused at the doorway of his partner's office. Derren Davide, a tall blond, blue-eyed Swede, had joined him last year, specializing in reconstruction with a focus on pediatric plastic surgery. Tate considered him a complement to his practice. He had charm and a vigorous dedication to medicine. At times, he thought Derren to be too imperious, but his patients loved him. His personal opinion of Derren had no place in business. Telling his impressions to Erin one evening, she surprised him when she said, "I'd watch my back if I were you."

Their only argument in their relationship might have been their last. He had come to expect little or no resistance to his opinions in recent years, but she challenged him, nudged him from his superior perch. In the end, he learned that winning an argument with an attorney took more energy than he wanted to spend, so he pretended to defer to her opinion to end the debate. She had plenty of exposure to the criminal classes, but he prided himself on being a better judge of character than she implied by warning him. Derren had impeccable references from his former hospitals. Still, he could not help wondering what Erin saw that he missed. He kept a vigilant eye on Derren since then that he would not have done otherwise.

"Good morning," Tate said.

Derren held up his hand, a signal between a wave and a stop gesture. "Can't talk now. I'm voting," and turned his eyes back to his computer screen.

Tate had listened *ad nauseum* to Derren's excitement

last week about participating in a local magazine competition for "Best Plastic Surgeon." Aside from having a medical degree, the magazine required each doctor pay for advertising space for inclusion in the roster of eligible physicians. Tate had told him he thought it was deceptive advertising and not a credible way to search for a doctor, but Derren disagreed.

"Listen, man," Derren had said, "This will bring in customers from the outlying areas of town. It's better than just advertising. To be the best in town according to an important magazine, well, that's gold."

"But, how can you be sure you'll win?"

"That's easy, everyone can vote once a day. I set up two hundred new emails. All I have to do is vote for me from each email every day until the end of the competition."

"Isn't that time consuming? What about your patients?"

"I'll do it every morning before the patients start coming. This is sure fire."

Tate thought but did not say that a doctor built a reputation through honest, hard work, like any other profession or trade, not by gimmicks and con games. Derren would not listen. So there he sat, sending his two hundred emails. The trouble with Derren's tactic was that another plastic surgeon seemed to have had the same idea. They were within a few votes of each other every day so far. A lot of effort for a valueless designation.

Tate shook his head and continued to his office. He closed his door, dropped into his desk chair, and stared out the window for several seconds before reaching for his cellphone. He scrolled through his address book, paused at Erin's photo, and pressed the send button to her cell.

"Hey," he said when she answered.

"Holding up alright today?

The warmth from her soft voice emanated through the line and enveloped him. "Not much better. I can't get past the shock that he's gone. I couldn't sleep last night for seeing him lying on that bed."

"If it makes you feel any better, I volunteered to represent Imogen," Erin said. "I remember the way she acted the other day. Once I speak with her, I'll know for certain, but I want her examined for competency if the District Attorney doesn't. While she was responsive, she seemed easily broken, like a child. My heart went out to her."

"Using the temporary insanity defense argument will make this a high-profile case. That's not going to hurt your career," he said. Tate knew this childish comeback did not become him, but he wanted her to sympathize with his perspective, not take the side of the woman who caused his loss.

"That's not fair."

"I'm sorry. Forget I said that. Listen, my first patient is due at nine. I need to go. Thanks for taking Imogen's case. I hope you can help her. I don't feel too charitable towards her right now, but I guess she needs representation as anyone would."

"Don't forget we're invited to the Bellows for dinner tonight." When he did not speak, she said, "I spoke with Lorraine this morning. They understand what you've just been through. We discussed whether to cancel, but we agreed that a good dinner with friends might be therapeutic for you. It doesn't have to be a long evening. Please say you'll go."

"My appointment's here. I have to go. We'll talk later." He disconnected the call feeling antagonistic. His blood boiled inside, but he had to set his emotions aside for the next few hours. No matter how he felt, he disciplined himself to remain neutral around his patients. They had their own problems. Some trauma patients had psychological and physical issues from the devastation of their injuries. He believed physicians should provide an environment that centered on the patients' needs and that patients should never perceive their doctor's mood. He took a deep breath when the intercom on his desk beeped.

"Mrs. Allen is here. I put her in Room Two."

Four breast reconstruction consultations, a browlift, a necklift, a nose job follow-up, and two tummy tuck pre-op appointments provided a temporary reprieve from his mourning. The focus on his work had done him good, but the pain crept back during the walk to his car. Any other distraction he tried to use to erase the images from the night before, the more he came back around to Henry. Henry had grown to be a bigger part of his life than he had acknowledged before this happened. He would miss him.

The Vines, pushed back in his mind all morning, crept back through visuals so vivid that they might have been real. At least now, the images were less intense as last night. He steadied his pace, and reflected how he dealt with trauma throughout his career. Clinical evaluation of the patient's physical damage, and then devise and execute a plan of action. But he had no game plan for dealing with emotional distress, his or anyone else's. He steered his attention to a welcome evening with Erin and the Bellows. Before he turned on the engine, he called Erin to tell her he would be there.

"It might do me good to be around people, but in case it gets to be too much, I want to be able to leave without ruining your evening. I'll meet you there."

"Hey, I don't mind. Whatever it takes. All we want is to be there for you."

"Don't think I don't appreciate the gesture. This thing has shaken me to my core. One minute I need to be alone, the next, I want to be inside a crowd. Being with my patients redirected my thoughts for a while."

"I'm glad you decided to go. By the way, I'm leaving my office now and heading over to meet with Imogen at the jail," Erin said. "Then, I'm taking a quick break to meet Hermione at my place for lunch before I go back to the office."

"I didn't know she was in town."

"She arrived early this morning for a short visit. She made a dinner appointment with a potential client here in Phoenix, and then she's off to Denver tomorrow evening for an afternoon appointment the next day. Since Denver's so close, she found that an excuse to have a quick visit. It's been over a year since we've been able to coordinate our schedules. I'll tell you all about it later. I'm glad you're feeling better. I've been worried about you. You can be too much your own island at times."

"I'll get past this. It's the shock of violence happening to someone you know. I didn't have a clue that..." He heard his voice crackle from unexpected emotion.

"I wish I could say something magical or profound to help. But you know that I'm here if you need to talk. I'll see you tonight."

He disconnected the call, belted, and reached to turn the ignition key. Fatigue rushed over him. He yawned and blinked several times to clear his vision, He tapped the gas pedal, ready to push down on the clutch and put in reverse, when he heard a tapping on his window. He saw Derren bent down and smiling at him, speaking before Tate had time to lower the window.

"I just heard about your friends. I'm sorry to hear it. Terrible experience for you. How are you doing?"

"As well as anyone can expect under the circumstances," Tate said.

"Let me know if I can do anything for you, Bud."

That nickname, Bud, annoyed the hell out of Tate, but he let it go. "Thanks. I will. I'm out for the rest of the day unless I'm called in on an emergency." He pressed the button that raised the window before Derren finished his last sentence.

Derren gave Tate's car a light pat to the roof and then a half salute when the car moved out of its space. Tate watched him from the rearview mirror and had what his grandmother called a twinge—a feeling in his gut trying to tell him to pay attention to something important. That happened whenever he talked to Derren. He had no clue what he needed to see. With all that had gone on with Imogen, he made the conscious choice to put other concerns on hold. For now. He put the car in gear, and moved forward to the exit gate. He hoped that choice would not bite him later.

CHAPTER THREE

Monica enjoyed the early November breeze blowing over her. She looked at the desert plants placed around the small tables of Her Majesty's Court, dubbed "The Court" by the locals. The waiter had brought her a glass of wine while she waited for her friends. She smiled considering how funny that she arrived ahead of the others whenever they got together, managing to greet them with the quirky smile, her first sign of intoxication.

She closed her eyes to take in the calming garden sounds before the girls arrived with the rest of the lunch rush. The peace of her surroundings had started to send her into a nap. She shot upright when she remembered the smudge marks mascara leaves on her under-eye area. She popped open her eyes and pulled out a small hand mirror to check. Safe for now, she thought. Behind her, she heard the approach of clicking heels.

Monica recognized Fleur's distinctive walk before she saw her, her stomping stiletto heels on the concrete floor in the bar, and then on the outside patio's wood deck planks. Monica turned her head to greet her when a couple passed Fleur on their way out. Monica noticed how Fleur made eye contact with the man and smiled, but disregarded the female accompanying him. She doubted Fleur would put up with that in the reverse situation.

"Hey, Chicky," Fleur said. She sat down next to Monica, and surveyed the few patrons at the other tables.

"Who are you looking for?"

"Just checking out the crowd for Mister Right," Fleur laughed. "Or at least, Mister Convenient. It's good to see you." She reached over to give Monica a pseudo cheek kiss before turning her attention to a table of suited men in serious conversation at the opposite end of the patio. "I heard the fundraising went well."

"I missed you there."

"You know me. I hate crowds, but I sent in a generous check to cover your disappointment."

Monica smiled. Fleur's audacious nerve amused her. She noted the young waiter approaching their table had an uneasy look, probably because this would not be his first encounter with the woman who made a sport out of seducing waiters. Nothing practical occurred to Fleur, like holding up her hand or waiting for their turn. Monica cringed at Fleur's flirtatious eye contact with every man she met. Monica guessed that was how Fleur learned how to get what she wanted. But it would be a mistake to typecast her. She had brains, courage, and fierce loyalty to her close friends, especially her female friends.

"Chardonnay, please, and another of whatever giggle juice my friend is drinking," Fleur said. Monica grinned at the fearful expression in the young man's face.

"I need to eat something soon or I'll be 'three sheets to the wind' by the time the others get here," Monica said. She wondered why she always worried about drinking wine before she ate, but did it anyway.

"What exactly does that mean? I've heard that all my life," Fleur said. "and I still don't understand how three bed sheets blowing on a clothesline have anything to do with being drunk."

"I'm not sure either, but it sounds better than *shit-faced*."

"Monica, not again!" Another familiar voice came from behind her, and she turned to see Devon Bateman. They had assigned Devon as their group's token blonde friend under forty.

"Not yet, but if I don't eat soon, I will be," Monica said. She stood to give her a full hug. Devon had an intrinsic sadness about her that brought out Monica's maternal protectiveness. Maybe the nine years' difference between them was significant, or maybe Devon wore a helpless nature like a subliminal calling card.

Once seated again, Monica sipped her wine and watched Fleur and Devon embrace. Monica tried to decide which woman was prettier. While Devon was blonde, blue-eyed, and fair—Fleur had light brown hair, peaches and cream complexion, and hazel eyes. Both around the same height and built small, their looks a startling contrast from the other, but both were stunning in their own right. Monica amused herself with the idea that she created a further contrast to them. Her dark brown hair and dark brown eyes exaggerated her distinct Latina appearance next to them. Devon's raised voice interrupted her thoughts.

"Frankie, you're here!"

While they went through the cordialities, Monica's gnawing sense of trouble returned as it did whenever she saw Frankie. Francesca Campbell, Frankie to friends, an attractive, confident, and successful restaurateur owned an elegant destination restaurant. She had built the business with her bare hands from the ground up with no help from anyone but her banker. Monica admired her ambition. With dark blonde hair, brown eyes, and sleek muscular body in a tight forty-six year old package,

Frankie had energy rivaling women half her age. Still, Monica sensed something furtive about her, an incongruity with her public image. Out of habit, she set those thoughts aside, stood, and gave Frankie a mock hug. "Mwah-mwah. Good to see you, Franks." Monica thought that deep down, she and Frankie had a mutual dislike of each other.

"So Monica, how's that hunky man you're sleeping with?"

"Frankie, who's been spreading rumors I sleep with men?" Monica said. "There's very little sleeping involved. And Troy is very fine, now that you ask."

Frankie raised her chin and looked away. "I swear, you and Fleur have had sex with more men this last year than I have my entire life. It's raunchy."

"Jealous much?" Monica stuck out her tongue, before she emptied her wine glass and raised it in the air to signal the waiter.

"I wish you wouldn't drag me into this," Fleur said. "Who cares, anyway?"

"What a beautiful day to sit outside," Devon said. "This time of year in Phoenix is intoxicating."

"I agree," Fleur said, "enough chill in the air to be refreshing without making you cold."

Monica looked to Frankie, a tinge of regret about her earlier thoughts. She should not let Frankie bait her that way. "How's the restaurant doing? This is the start of your busy season, isn't it?"

"Sure is," Frankie said. "I was in at six this morning to make sure the orders were set up. Then I had to find replacements for the busboy and the hostess, who it turns out, are sleeping together. They both called in to say their car stalled in Flagstaff. What a pain in the ass. Luke was in by nine and took over. I don't know what I'd do without him."

"You need a glass of wine," Monica said.

"No, not for me today. I have to keep a clear head. Too much to do. I was just telling Dr. Tate about my schedule this morning."

"Another Botox appointment so soon?" Fleur said.

"No. I was in for a consultation about a brow lift."

"A browlift!" Monica said. "Does he think you need one?"

"Not really, but he said he would do it if I wanted," Frankie said.

"That doesn't sound like him. Isn't he usually resistant to doing unnecessary surgeries?"

"Monica, *dear*, he would do it because I wanted it. Anyway, he showed me pictures of other women who've had browlifts by him. Don't mention a word, but showing me those photos is a big no-no, but he knows he can trust me."

"Frankie, *dearest*, did you drop acid this morning?" Monica said. "Why would Dr. Tate bend his ethics for you? Or anyone, for that matter? Anyway, we all signed disclosures about photos. Remember? He's not showing you anything he shouldn't."

Devon and Fleur looked from one to the other in tennis-match style, eyes going from Frankie to Monica and back again. "And if you believe he did something wrong, why are you talking about it with all the ears around us?"

"I mentioned it because I thought you could all be trusted."

Monica blinked her eyes and looked at Frankie. "Okay, *Lady of Shalott.* If you say so." Monica decided it was time to change the subject. "I didn't tell you the best part of the fundraiser. When the Judge made a comment that we needed more plastic surgeons like Dr. Tate, Imogen looked at him and said she thought he said he was a gynecologist. Something like that. You know how Imogen thinks she's the funniest woman living. Well, she started laughing like a hyena while the rest of us waited to see how Tate would react. Eventually, he started to laugh after Erin said something in his ear."

"Oh my gosh. Did she really say that?" Devon said. "She always says she finds herself amusing. Too bad no one else does." Devon chuckled. "Hey, where is she, anyway?"

"She was in a funny mood the other night. I think she and Henry had been fighting," Monica said. "Whatever the problem, she acted very weird. I took her home and gave her space. She'll call one of us when she's ready."

Frankie pulled her cell phone from the outside pocket of her purse, pushed a couple of buttons, and put the phone to her ear. In response to the others questioning looks, she said, "I'm calling Imogen. See if she wants to join us."

After a minute, she started to talk in monotone message voice, "Hey, Girl. We're at the Court missing you. There's still time to join us if you're free. Call me." When she hung up, she looked around the table with an odd expression and said, "I hope she's all right."

After lunch, Frankie drove home and poured a large whiskey. In an uncharacteristic indulgence, she turned on the television to watch the news. When she saw a photo of Imogen and Henry flash across the screen, she paused and rewound to listen to the news story. She had heard right. Henry Vine dead. Imogen Vine in jail for killing him. Tate Marsdon found the body. Erin Fitzgerald to defend Imogen.

"Tragic and disturbing," the newscaster said.

She only hoped that Imogen would keep her secret. The last thing Frankie needed was for her to blab her confidences to strangers.

Frankie twisted her hands, unsure what she should do next. *He* must know what happened by now. She dreaded telling him she had shared his *indiscretions* to Imogen. If she were lucky, Imogen would be too preoccupied with her own problems to spill her secret. He would be furious either way. He might even hit her again, or dump her for good this time. The reporter talked like Imogen had snapped and was incapable of having a lucid conversation with anyone. All Frankie could hope for now was for Imogen's fog to become permanent. Would that be enough to satisfy him? Or would he want to make sure she never remembered?

She eyed the decanter for a few seconds before deciding to have another drink. *To hell with the restaurant today.* Her shaking hands created jiggling waves inside the glass as she poured. When she sat again, she spotted the bottle of leftover Valium on the kitchen counter. She knew that was a bad idea, but the more she considered her frayed nerves, the better a tranquilizer sounded. She carried her drink to the kitchen, took out a tiny blue pill from the bottle, and washed it down with a large volume of whiskey. Her throat stung. "Yow! I guess there's a reason you're not supposed to gulp hard liquor."

Satisfied that would calm her jittery nerves, she walked to the living room sofa, and grabbed her cell phone before falling into the deep cushions. She thought of whom she could call for help concerning Imogen. She had to find a friend who would interpret her curiosity as concern for Imogen, and not question her motives. "Aha," she said. "Monica." She was a bit of a smart ass, but most of that was bluster. When Monica hears Imogen's trouble, she won't become suspicious that this is more than worry over a friend.

Monica cringed when she noticed their late lunch lasted until after five. She stayed behind and drank several cups of coffee before leaving to run errands prior to going home, but she still had a light buzz. She took her time driving north on Central Avenue, her favorite section of road in Phoenix. The row of the mature Arizona Ash trees that canopied over the road gave her the feeling of being in the east where trees were so tall that they created a tunnel effect. She turned east on Lawrence on her way to pick up a donation bag from an elderly lady from church, when she heard her cell phone and pulled over to answer it.

Monica sensed a doom rush over her when she saw Frankie's face flashing on the phone. She gave out a moan before she answered. "Hello." She anticipated a continuation of their earlier conversation at the Court, but prodded herself to keep an open mind and to be civil. *Wait to hear what Frankie has to say before you condemn her.*

"I've just learned the most horrible news," Frankie said.

"My God, what is it?"

"Imogen killed Henry! Not only did she kill him, but she also lived with his corpse for three days. That means when you were out with her, Henry was lying dead in the house the whole time." Frankie's voice grew higher with every word until she started sobbing. Monica's mind drew visions of the histrionics of a Vaudeville stage performer.

"Frankie, where are you?"

"At...home," she said through sobs.

"I'll be right over. Have a drink or a Valium. I'll be there in ten."

Monica continued up Lawrence, turned left onto Third Street and right onto Glendale Road until it turned into Lincoln Drive. Monica drove without seeing the traffic or knowing how she got there. Before she started to pay attention, she had pulled in front of Frankie's two-story ranch-cum-colonial east of the Phoenix boundary in Paradise Valley.

She shrugged off her shock at the news about Imogen for a minute while she cursed out loud at her irritation of Frankie's gravel driveway. Marveling, as she had done before, that what use was making all that frickin' money when you could not pave your driveway? She stepped onto the gravel and felt her stiletto sink through the gravel down to the dirt. She cringed as she heard the sharp edges scratch at her heels. Her black Lexus SUV that had been shiny and clean now looked like she had taken it through a dust storm or had gone off-roading. Yes, this was irrelevant to the bigger issue, but she took one more pained look at her vehicle anyway before schlepping on tiptoes to the front door.

Frankie peered out before she opened the door to let Monica enter. Nothing looked changed as far as Monica could see, especially the liquor cabinet to the left of the foyer with its doors flung wide open. Monica's eyes followed the room's contour to the sunken living room where a tall glass of something amber swirled around melting ice cubes. She saw a small prescription bottle sitting open next to its cap. Monica, braced for drama, turned around to face Frankie, who looked visibly shaken.

"How did you hear about this? I would think there'd be something on the news before now."

"Well, it's on the news now, but they're keeping most of the details secret," Frankie said. "Either the police are withholding, or it's because Henry and Imogen were well-connected and had many friends in the press. But, good God, how could she do such a thing?"

"Probably during one of their ridiculous arguments."

"No, not the killing-him part—that I understand. I mean how could she live with a dead body for three days? Murder is easy. Living with a dead man, now that's insane. I never took Imogen to be crazy."

"Me either, but people snap," Monica said. "You know yourself how cruel couples can be to each other."

"Still, I can't believe it. Imogen was fine last week when we met for breakfast."

"Did you take a Valium with your bourbon," Monica said. "You look stoned."

"Yes, but I needed it. I've had a great shock. Poor Imogen. I guess they'll have her meeting with every kind of psychiatrist, ask her dozens of questions about the days leading up to the event, and ask her to describe living with a corpse in her bed. I'm scared for her."

Monica thought how far Frankie had thought all this through. She knew Frankie and Imogen were close friends, but she had not imagined Frankie caring about anyone so much to cause her to lose her rigid composure. Frankie, the poster girl for the motivated narcissist, calculated every step in her life for a particular aim. To see this unemotional woman transforming into an empathetic person brought to mind the pods in *Invasion of the Body Snatchers*. Except here, a human emerged to replace the creature.

"Come sit down with me." Frankie motioned Monica into the living room. "We need to figure out what to do."

"All I can think to do is to call the police station and

ask about her status. I think her kids are in other states. I've never known their names, much less how to get in touch. They were an independent couple with lots of interest. They didn't share much about their children."

"Well, call the damn police! We have to know what's going on."

Monica had to make the effort to close her dropped jaw. "Frankie, how many Valium have you taken?"

"I've had just the one Valium and two whiskey chasers. Why do you ask?"

"No reason. Give me your phone?" Monica grabbed it from her and dialed the Crime Stop number she knew by heart.

While Frankie poured another drink, Monica spoke to someone on the other end of the line and found out that Imogen was in custody, held without bail. After a few more minutes of listening, Monica disconnected the call and turned to Frankie, who had popped another Valium in her mouth.

"Well, that's interesting. Do you remember I told you about Dr. Tate's girlfriend at the reception? She's going to represent Imogen. Isn't that great? The cop also said her lawyer filed court documents requesting a mental-competency exam. At least, that's something."

Frankie took a sip and said, "I saw that on the news. Why the 'ef' is she sticking her nose into this situation?"

"Frankie, I'm surprised at you. I assume that she heard about the trouble and thought she could help. Somebody's got to defend poor Imogen. Isn't it better that it's someone we kind of know something about?"

"Yes, but why *her*, of all people?"

"Is there something you're not telling me, because what I know about her is she has a good standing in the legal community. She's won so many impossible cases the press compares her to Perry Mason. Besides, Dr. Tate has been the Vines' friend for years. I'd think he'd step in if he believed Erin was not the right lawyer for her."

"When you put it that way," Frankie said. "I guess you're right."

Monica watched Frankie sink into her overstuffed chair with a groan, and wondered if she knew Frankie as well as she thought she did. Her behavior was over-the-top weird considering Imogen was the one in trouble.

"Listen, Frankie. Maybe you should try to sleep this off. You're making me nervous. I'm going to go down to the police station and see if I can get in to see Imogen. They probably won't let me, but they might give her a message that I came. I want her to know I support her."

Frankie shifted to lean on the sofa arm, and said, "You're right. I'm just upset. Go see what you can find out, and let me know, will you?"

"I will. I'll call when I learn something," Monica said. She closed the door behind her, and got in her car. Getting the full concentration of Frankie on her own today made her uneasy. Or maybe it was the creep factor of the circumstances. Two close friends had transformed into different women in one day, confirming the adage that no one can ever really know another person.

When Erin arrived back at her office, Penny Lykens smiled. "Nice lunch?"

Penny knew her well enough to recognize her stress.

"Yes, I did, as a matter of fact, but we're back in the game. Get me a number for Monica Aames and find out if she's available tomorrow morning. She's a friend of Imogen Vine. She might be able to shed some light on a couple of things. I don't feel I'm getting through to

Imogen. She doesn't remember me, so I need to find out how to earn her trust, if that's even possible."

Penny smiled at the last comment. She watched Erin until she closed her office door behind her. She admired Erin's talent for persistence, but also her show business attitude that the show must go on. Not more apparent than now after what her boyfriend went through.

Monica finished her workout, and noticed the red message light flashing on her phone. Good, she thought. Business had been slow the last year. Not a lot of calls for fundraising event organizers. Even during the good times, she felt like a bottom feeder taking money from charities. Now, with some non-profits barely scraping by due to reduced funding from the government sector, she had pressure to work free, but she had to live. Not to mention covering the thousands she spent upfront that went into organizing each event.

She brought her breathlessness to a professional tone and said, "Monica Aames."

"Ms. Aames, this is Penny Lykins from Erin Fitzgerald's office. She would like to arrange a meeting with you concerning Imogen Vine's defense. She has concerns and feels a good friend might give her insight into Mrs. Vine's life and personality."

"Of course, anything I can do to help. When did you have in mind?"

"How's tomorrow morning at ten?"

"That's no problem. I'm available."

"That's great. What about other close friends? Anyone else you think might be helpful?"

"Yes, that would be Frankie Campbell, Devon Bateman, and Fleur Sanders. We've been close for many years. I can call them, if that helps. Find out if they're free and invite them."

"That's very helpful. Erin will be pleased. See you tomorrow at ten. Her office is downtown. Here's the address."

She typed the details into her phone calendar, and carried her gear to the showers. None of this seemed real, more like walking through a dream waiting to wake up and escape the distorted landscape of the real world.

CHAPTER FOUR

By the time he and Erin had seated themselves at the dinner table with the Bellows, Tate's tension and fatigue had started to wear through his personal armor. From the time he drove out of the garage at work, his bad feelings had grown disproportionately. He blamed Derren, between his impromptu encounter in the parking garage and the anxiety over his skewed professionalism. Those nagging worries compounded by his grief and shock over the Vines. His mind looped in a vicious cycle between worry and horror.

After a drink, a nap, and a shower, he had developed a headache instead of feeling refreshed. He convinced himself that he could handle a social evening, but could he? What had he been thinking that sitting down to a civilized meal as if nothing had happened might relax him? When he watched Erin receiving the salutary hug from Lorraine at the door, he admitted he came because he had not wanted to disappoint her. He drew in a breath, took the offered drink, and looked over to Lorraine making a point about the Caribbean to her husband.

"I always thought the Caribbean would be magical. Instead, I found the contrast between rich and poor to be more marked than even here in the States. I'm too sensitive and empathetic to enjoy myself in that environment," Lorraine said "knowing how those people work all day in luxurious surroundings, then go home to decaying buildings and poverty."

Eyeing her with amusement, the judge looked at his wife with loving antagonism. While they openly challenged each other on every subject imaginable, any observer could see how much they adored each other. With a slight chuckle, he turned to her and said, "My dear, some countries are better at hiding their social inequities than others, but that doesn't mean they don't exist. Remember that if not for the tourist trade, these same people would have no income." His salt and pepper goatee and light grey eyes gave him an authoritarian bearing, sure to have helped him in his role as judge imparting justice from the bench. Whether that helped him in his bantering with Lorraine was another matter.

Lorraine glanced in Tate's direction with a questioning look, and then over to Erin sitting across from him. "Have you two been to any of the islands?"

Erin cleared her throat and said, "No I haven't. I've always wanted to but I've been too busy going to school and working the last several years. What about you, hon?"

My queue, he thought. I'm expected to do small talk. "Same for me. My parents took us to Europe several summers when I was a boy, but I don't remember much of those trips." He felt their eyes on him and knew they were trying to be delicate. "I know you're all curious about what happened to the Vines. If you want to talk about it, I don't mind. It's a tragedy and a horrible waste of two lives, but there's not much I can do about it."

"I can't imagine how you feel. But, please let us know how we can help you through this. Don't hesitate for a second," Lorraine said. She reached out and laid her hand on his forearm.

Tate smiled at her before looking at Erin who wiped

the corners of her mouth with her napkin and took a sip of wine. He thought she might be trying to look invisible in this conversation.

"You might not have heard yet, but Erin has signed on to defend her." He struggled to make his tone even and forced a weak smile.

"You're going to plead temporary insanity, I assume. That will be difficult to support, depending on her current state of mind," Barry said. "Have you spoken with her yet?"

"Briefly, without any luck though. I don't believe she's faking. From what I can see, she has disconnected from the event and doesn't understand where she is. She started mumbling about a girl and how sad about what happened. No one knows what she's talking about either, so this could be a delusion. If this continues, she won't get to the point of standing trial. I'll know more after her psych evaluation."

"What a delicate woman, but we underestimate the fragile ones, don't we?" Lorraine said, staring into her wine glass.

Listening to this conversation made Tate lightheaded. He noticed his three dinner companions sneaking glances to check on his reactions, he guessed. After what he considered a respectable time after dinner, he put his napkin on the table and looked over to Lorraine, "I have to leave. The truth is I misjudged the effects this experience has had on me. I'll feel better getting home to bed."

"No dessert?" Lorraine leaned over, tilted her head in his direction. "Well, we understand. We appreciate you coming over this evening."

"Absolutely, young man," Barry said. "It's not easy losing a friend, especially by someone else's hand. Two lives absolutely destroyed, not to mention the impact on their children, friends, and associates. Remember that you're a victim, too."

"It's going to take time before I get rid of this sickening feeling," Tate said. "Working with anonymous cadavers in school doesn't compare to seeing your friend dead in front of you."

"Would you like company this evening? I can meet you at your place," Erin said.

"I'm not up to it. I think I'll be better on my own," Tate said. "Besides, Hermione is waiting for you. You two need to catch up. I'll be fine." He stood up and left after a hug from Lorraine, a handshake with Barry, and a gentle kiss on Erin's cheek. He leaned into her ear and whispered, "Say hello to Hermione for me."

After they heard the click of the closing front door, Barry looked to Erin. "He needs to work things out on his own. Maybe he'll change his mind and get therapy. Being a judge for so long, I've seen too many human casualties. The innocent bystanders to crime, the witnesses, the neighbors, the children of murder victims, and murderer's families, suffer life-altering emotional scars that imprint them for life. They're the least thought of, too."

"I wonder how long this kind of thing will affect him," Erin said. "He seems so disturbed, so broken. I'm frightened for him."

Barry shifted in his seat, took a drink, and said, "It's like the follow-up story I read in the paper this morning about that young girl who was strangled and left for dead in the parking garage at Sky Harbor. The police said they're attempting to track the owners of the vehicles that left around the estimated time of death, but that's not an easy task. Not like on television, when they run a couple of facts through an impressive computer and get five viable suspects within two minutes. They're scanning the security camera footage, but her vehicle was just out of range."

"That figures," Lorraine said.

"Whoever killed her must have had an idea of where the cameras were and how to avoid them. It's tragic for her parents. She was an only child, a brilliant scholar in her first year of medical school. My point here is that every violent death affects many people, from the one who found her to her family and friends, even occasional acquaintances."

"True," Erin said. "That happened around two weeks ago, right?"

"Yes," Lorraine said. "I remember so well because we had arrived at the airport that afternoon from Laguna Beach. When I heard the story on the news, I thought how scary to think we might have seen the murderer without knowing. You remember, darling, when I said what a coincidence so many people we knew were at the airport at the same time?"

Barry laughed, "I got a kick out of that, because we saw Derren and Tate passing us from the long-term parking garages in different cars. We joked about their timing after the news came out."

"That's when they went to the medical convention in Las Vegas." Erin smiled with them. "Still, the poor girl. I wonder who killed her. It might turn out the police never catch the guy. It does happen, as incredible as that is to realize."

"The article hinted that the police have leads, but they're withholding certain facts from the public," Barry finished his wine, his eyes peering over the glass at Erin.

"We don't need any more shock-and-awe stories from the press who'll print anything for ratings—true or not."

Before Erin could continue, Lorraine stood up abruptly. "Let's get our minds off of death for a while. I'll get dessert and coffee ready, and we can relax in the living room."

As they drank coffee, ate crème brûlée, and chatted about trivialities in front of the large fireplace that hosted a roaring flame, Erin hid her real thoughts behind polite conversation, as she guessed her companions did. Erin wondered what the Bellows thought of Imogen and Henry, and what the Judge saw as the inevitable verdict on Imogen. What she wondered more was whether the judge thought she was up to the task of defending his friend, which had the potential to taint the memory of Henry, a friend unable to defend himself?

Erin looked forward to seeing Hermione, her friend who knew her better than anyone. Her visit will be a refuge from the trouble. An opportunity to retreat into the innocent days of high school again, even if for a short time.

Erin walked into her apartment to find Hermione watching television.

"Hermione Jones. Am I ever glad you're here," Erin said. She dumped her purse and jacket, and went over to embrace her friend.

"This is like high school. Hanging out with nothing to do but watch television, except without the drugs, eh?"

"I wouldn't want to relive those days," Erin said.

"Me either. So how's everything? I saw the story about Tate on the news. I'd be a wreck if that happened to me.

I'd have nightmares the rest of my life."

"No kidding. I think he's going to be fine, but it's early days. He's still processing and trying to cope. He's intellectual and analytical, so I see him trying to make sense of what happened, and then reconcile how two people he admired could end up that way."

"You know," Hermione said. "I've always said we're all capable of murder, but for most of us our moral filters kick in before we act on our impulses."

"I saw Imogen on Saturday at the fundraiser. She acted strange but I thought she had a bad case of nerves about her speech. She's attractive and charming, but not a substantial intellect."

"So, you're going to defend her? What's that like? There's no question she did it. You specialize in the circumstantial cases, don't you?"

"Yes, but I thought I would do what I could for her considering she's Tate's friend."

"Ah-hah! Brownie points for the boyfriend," Hermione said, jabbing Erin's ticklish waist with her forefinger.

Erin blushed. "So what! Someone has to defend her. She doesn't know criminal attorneys, and the ones Henry used for business haven't volunteered. Besides, I doubt this will take much time. From my brief conversation with her, she seems to be out of touch with reality. She didn't recognize me."

"You don't think he'll be mad if the case doesn't go that way? I mean, would he be mad if she's found not guilty?"

"I hope not. I've done the deed so there's no turning back now. By the way, did you have dinner with the client?"

"I met him, but he didn't have time for dinner. I had a

drink and an appetizer. I was anxious to get here, so I took a taxi here and took my chances you'd have food. I had a crunchy peanut butter sandwich, and finished off your Cheetos with the wine while I watched a movie. I'm good."

"I don't have much in the line of breakfast food, so why don't we go out in the morning and get a bite before I go to the office. I have a couple of appointments, and then I'll pick you up for a late lunch. We can play the rest of the day," Erin said. Hermione did not try to hide her disappointment.

"I won't be gone long. I promise. It's another new client, then a quick visit with Imogen."

"I understand. I dropped in with only a day's notice. It's just that as we get older, I feel life slipping by me. I'll be working or doing anything, and then I feel an urgency to see you, as if I have to enjoy your company as much as I can before I lose the opportunity. Sometimes I get scared."

Erin teared up, and reached over to hug her. "I get those feelings too. It's our age and knowing what's to come. When we were goofy teenagers, we had our whole lives in front of us like there was no mistake we couldn't undo. Now, we know our limitations. But let's focus on the now and stop wondering about the indefinable future. We'll be having this conversation when we're eighty."

"You're right. I guess I should stop drinking wine. I get too emotional. Knowing alcohol is a depressant doesn't seem to put things in perspective."

"Stop being serious. Have more wine and tell me what man brought on this gloom."

CHAPTER FIVE

Monica joined the others in the front lobby at Erin's law office. She took turns watching her friends, finding the seriousness of the situation affected each of them differently. Frankie had the expression of someone about to be executed. Devon sat upright in her chair, looking out of the tall windows that overlooked downtown Phoenix. Fleur, on the other hand, seemed unaffected, surveying the furnishings or her nail polish, checking her phone for messages. Monica had sat in many law offices over the years to attend organizational meetings for her charity clients. For her, the environment had little to influence her mood.

When Penny Lykins finally came out, all four of them tensed up. Monica could not help but flash back on visits to the principal's office after getting busted for smoking. They walked single-file into a large meeting room.

"Have a seat anywhere you're comfortable. There's coffee, tea, and water in the kitchenette. Help yourselves. Ms. Fitzgerald will be right in. She's finishing up a phone call."

"Thank you," Monica said. The others said nothing, but poured coffee and chose a seat.

Monica saw Erin walking down the hall from her office. She hesitated, took a deep breath, and opened the door. Brisk and professional, definitely wearing her lawyer hat today. She had been less formal when they met at the party, but even then, in that casual environment, Monica saw the starch in her manner.

"Good morning, ladies. Thank you for coming on short notice. As Imogen's friends, I know you're anxious to help her. As you might or might not know, Imogen has suffered a sort of break with reality. Her recollection of recent events is spotty. She has no memory of Henry's death. One problem we're having is she has a high level anxiety over a young girl."

"What young girl?" Monica leaned in closer. "What's this new twist?

"That's the problem. Imogen doesn't remember. She's so vague that she has no idea who I am at present. Tate doesn't recall either of them mentioning an incident involving a girl. I wondered if the girl might be one of their daughters, or a niece. I hoped one of you might be able to help. If we could relieve her concerns about this person, we might be able to move forward with her recovery."

Fleur spoke first. "I don't know that Imogen knows any young girls socially, maybe mothers of young girls."

"I've never heard her mention anyone, either," Devon said.

"Me either, but the last time I saw her, she had already…broken down," Monica said. Recalling that night gave her shivers when she thought that poor Henry was lying dead, a rotting corpse, while they were out having a good time.

The four women looked at Frankie who had not spoken since entering the room.

"Don't look at me," she said. "I don't know anything."

"Don't be so defensive. No one's accusing you of withholding information, for crying out loud," Monica said. "You and Imogen have been close in the past. It's natural we would ask you."

"I don't know anything about a young girl. If she's lost touch with reality, she probably picked up on something she heard on television and thinks it's real."

"That's possible," Erin said. Monica thought she looked disappointed. "I want you to know that I'm doing and will continue to do everything for her that's possible. She's not faking this loss of memory. It's common from what the psychiatrist tells me. The District Attorney has agreed that she needs treatment before a trial is possible. He's not worried. She did confess, and she's in custody in the hospital where she can't take off, or do herself harm."

"Can we see her?" Devon said.

"I'm afraid not yet. Later, the doctor may feel seeing you could assist him in her treatment. Seeing too many people too soon may confuse her and cause a setback. I don't know that she will recognize you, anyway. She's pretty vague on a lot of points."

"What happens now?" Fleur said.

Erin sighed. "Well, I visit her every day. Dr. Davenport sees her twice a day to work on her memory. He tells me that in cases like this, the fact that her attorney is someone she knows, whether she remembers me right now or not, can be beneficial. Seeing me might spark a memory, even the slightest thing, like recalling a necklace or scarf. Once she starts remembering, she'll be more likely to talk freely than if I were a stranger."

"Thank God you took her case," Monica said. "I don't mean to be personal, but isn't this awkward for you with Tate? He and Henry were like father and son."

Erin hesitated. Monica recognized the thought process behind the pause—the caution of a diplomatic mind. *Didn't Tate do that, too?* "I took on Imogen's case before I told him. He understands. It's just going to take time to heal."

"It's good of you to defend her," Monica said.

"Everyone deserves a good defense, even if they confess. It can mean a difference in the sentencing."

Monica looked at her friends. No one made a move to speak, so she said, "Please call us if Imogen needs anything. We want to help, but we don't know what to do."

"That's good to know. I'll keep you informed, as much as I can, of course." Erin smiled. "Thanks for taking time to come in. I appreciate your support."

Erin left the room, but they did not move right away.

"Well, I guess that's that." Monica stood up and the others followed her to the elevator.

"I wish we could've been more help," Devon said. "This whole thing is so messed up."

Frankie stared down at the carpet. "I wish I could see her, talk to her. I feel so helpless."

"We all do, Frankie," Monica said.

"All I can add," Fleur said, "is that if you're going to be tried for murder, you can't do any worse than having Erin represent you. Do you know she's never lost a case? They say she's like a pit bull when it comes to protecting her clients and finding out the truth. If we're lucky, she'll find out exactly what happened. Wouldn't it be great if Imogen turned out to be innocent?"

"It must be wonderful to live in that fantasy world of yours," Frankie said.

CHAPTER SIX

Hermione took advantage of the temperate weather, half walking, half jogging through Erin's neighborhood, the Alvarado Historic District. She caught her breath pausing to admire the stately Mission and Spanish Revival homes, lush green lawns, and wrought iron balconies. She ran down every street between Palm Lane and Oak, and Central and Third Street until she felt confident she had seen every home. Now she understood why Erin lived downtown.

She ran out of water during her sightseeing, and arrived back at the apartment parched and chalky. When she saw the bottled waters on the doormat outside the door, Hermione could not believe her luck. Erin must have dropped these off during her run. She twisted off the cap and drank it down as she made her way to the kitchen.

Getting close to lunchtime, her mid-section started to rumble. She finished off the first water and opened a second while she leaned into the refrigerator to survey the sparse contents of Erin's inventory. Hungry from missing a mid-morning snack, she thought how energizing it would be to have a little nibble before Erin got back. Not to her surprise, Erin had the essentials like eggs, bread, milk, and butter, but nothing prepackaged that she could gobble up fast. She found the same depressing results in the pantry. She thought a few seconds before settling on a drink to take the edge off her hunger.

She found gin and tonic in Erin's hallway cupboard in a makeshift liquor cabinet, and poured herself a double shot followed by the sparkling water. Before taking a drink, she thought of a lime in the fridge door. She set it on the cutting board and sliced it into thick slivers. *This qualifies as food.* She smiled and plopped one into the glass, and rubbed its juice around the rim with another. She added ice-cubes, stirred with her finger, and went to the patio outside the kitchen with a *Paris Match* magazine from the airport.

Not a warm day but a comfortable temperature for early afternoon, Hermione stared out onto the tops of palm trees in the area. While she had criticized Erin's choice to live downtown at first, she had learned what her friend saw in the area with its mature landscape, architecturally distinct home styles, no cookie-cutout developments here. Then, considering the nightlife, the culture, the pedestrian lifestyle, the area had the same personality as their childhood neighborhood in Philadelphia. Experience the ambiance without the weather that went with living in the East.

The soft breeze blew through her hair. She finished her gin and tonic, and then emptied her third water bottle. Stay hydrated. She decided on another drink, a decision that had always been a problem. The drink filled her up and satisfied her hunger, but she found it difficult to stop at one. What did it matter this time of day when she had nowhere important to be? Erin would drive. It was her turn, anyway. Hermione returned to her seat on the patio with a fresh drink. Days like this were what made Phoenix a treat in the winter months. "I could die happy sitting here looking at this view."

Hermione held up the French magazine, flipping past

the text that she did not understand. Reading made her drowsy, and she had started to nod off when she felt an overwhelming nausea and sharp pains deep inside her body. Her agonized yell interrupted the peace of the afternoon. She bent over as a reflex to comfort her mid-section, her body now trembling and sweating.

She burst through the patio door, and ran into the bathroom at the end of the hallway to throw up. Her skin grew numb and cold. She could not breathe. Concentrate. Think of what to do. The terrifying knowledge overtook her that she drank something toxic. Panic, regret, anger, helplessness, and guilt. How would Erin cope? She resisted until the violent attack overtook her. She collapsed at the bathroom door, deceived by a pause in the pain. Her lungs tightened into one last breath with a fitful gasp.

Erin smiled across at Imogen thinking that she expected Imogen to look more distraught. The psychiatrist had not made his evaluation yet, but she was confident the system would go easy on Imogen whatever that outcome. Delicate, fragile Imogen looked like a wilted flower removed from its vase too soon. Before a judge, jury, prosecutor and potential courtroom attendees, Imogen was a sympathetic figure who had endured the trauma of breast cancer and the subsequent surgeries. Still Erin doubted anyone could find that justification for coldblooded murder. She had no delusions that this case would go easy. Imogen had acted with "present ability" when she lied about Henry's whereabouts, used the dead animal deodorizer, and even kept the dinner invitation with Tate.

Imogen blinked as if she were trying to figure out who

she faced. "Don't I know you? I thought I was meeting my lawyer."

"We met several months ago at a restaurant with one of my clients. You introduced me to Tate."

Imogen brightened, and then massaged her temples. "Tate. Yes, something I need to tell him. Why can't I remember?"

Erin thought she was losing her. "Imogen, I volunteered to represent you. You didn't have an attorney. I believe I can help. Is that all right with you?"

"Sure. I don't know what you can do. I know I killed him. She told me I did. Everybody knows by now. What is there for you to do?"

"I know you've said you did it, but there's still a question of your state of mind, your health, if you were under any type of psychological stresses, that kind of thing."

"I see. I think. Memories come and go. I know there's something important I need to remember, but it keeps slipping away."

"Something to do with Henry?"

"I'm not sure," Imogen said. Her eyes lowered to study her hands.

Erin smiled. Oh boy, she thought. This might be more difficult than she anticipated if Imogen already drifted off into irrelevant areas when they were alone. Unpredictability in her behavior had the potential to blow up in their faces in court. She had to figure out how to get Imogen to focus when they talked.

"Imogen, listen to me. I've asked the court to refer your case to the Forensic Services Division to have you evaluated by doctors. Do you understand that?"

"I'm due for my follow-up appointment with Dr. Tate. Is that who's coming?"

Erin blinked. "No, not him. A different doctor who's going to talk to you about what happened with Henry and to make sure you're okay. We want to make sure you understand your situation."

"What's my situation?"

Chills ran down Erin's back. Imogen did not behave like someone who understood her situation. Either she sat across from a great actress or this woman had lost contact with reality.

"You're in jail. You've been arrested for killing Henry. Do you remember that?"

With a smug tolerance, Imogen looked at Erin and smiled, "That's ridiculous. I don't have a violent bone in my body. Ask anyone. I think you've confused me with that other woman."

Other woman? Where did that come from? Erin considered that pressing her into recalling the event might be harmful. Better to leave that for the doctor. He would know the best way to interact with her.

"Imogen, I'm going now. Is there anything I can bring you?"

"I'm worried about her and that girl's family. I said I would help, but I don't seem to be able to remember what I'm supposed to do."

"I'm sure everyone will understand, Imogen. You have the love and support from your friends and family. I've spoken to your kids. They're behind you no matter what, even if they can't get here."

"I don't blame them for not coming. Okay. I want to take a nap, so you'll have to go."

"That's not a problem." Erin reached into her purse, took out a business card, and pressed it in Imogen's hand.

"Keep this. Call me if you need anything at all."

Imogen looked at the card with passive curiosity. "I

don't expect I'll need it, but thanks for the thought."

Gesturing to the guard that she was ready to go, Erin and Imogen both stood. Erin fought the urge to hug her and left quickly. She looked back at Imogen through the small window in the door. A frightening vision of a woman lost inside herself. She would make a personal call to each of the women from the meeting this morning. Maybe one of them had been too embarrassed to speak in front of the others. Someone had to know something about this concern over a girl.

She tried Hermione's cell phone. No answer. She left a message that she was on her way home and looked forward to spending time with her again. "Ten minutes from the Madison Street Jail," she said in the voice message and disconnected. *Normality is what I need right now.*

Marguerite turned the key in the lock, and used her hip to shove open Erin's front door. She picked up her carryall crammed with cleaning supplies and walked inside. This was an easy job. The lady was neat and organized and never left a mess. Dusting, vacuuming, and cleaning the bathrooms. That was the job. In and out in an hour.

When she walked into the kitchen to set up, she saw the open patio door and froze. Had there been a break-in? Could the burglar still be here? She stopped to listen for movement, but heard nothing. She rallied, pulled out a chef's knife from the rack, and inched her way to the patio. Keeping an eye on the inside of the apartment, she pulled out her cell phone from her pocket and dialed 911.

"I got to my job and found the patio door open. The lady who lives here is very careful about locking up, so I think someone broke in. He might still be here."

"Give me the address," the dispatcher said.

Marguerite whispered the address.

"Stay on the line with me until the officers get there. They should arrive in a couple of minutes."

"Okay." Marguerite stood in the middle of the balcony, anxious to see a squad car moving her way, but afraid to take her eyes off the inside of the apartment. She wished she had something clever to say, but nothing came to her. Instead, she stood motionless, repeating, "Uh-huh" when asked if she were still there.

She heard a car pull up in front of the building. Relieved to see a police car, she waved down to them. In another minute, they were at the door, moving through the living room, the kitchen, and then the hallway. That is when she heard one officer say, "We have a body." The words pierced Marguerite. Poor Erin. Not her. She was so full of life.

"Marguerite?"

She jumped at the sound of her name. She looked up at the fair complexion of one of the officers. "Yes?"

"Did you go into the hall when you got here?"

"No, I went to the kitchen to set down my cleaning supplies. That's when I noticed the patio door open," she said. "I came out here to call the police and stayed on this spot to wait."

"Please stay here. We've found a female body in the hall. Brown hair, tall, slender, light skin. Does that sound like the woman who lives here?"

Marguerite sighed. "No. Erin has long auburn hair. Thank God, she's okay."

"Do you have any idea who she is," the officer said.

"No, sir. Unless it's someone visiting from out of town. I don't know her friends. I just come to clean every week. That's it."

"Do you have a cell number for Erin?"

"Yes, sir," she said. She scrolled through her cell phone contact list. She held the phone out so he could read the number. "She's going to be upset when she finds out about this. It's bad enough dealing with crime at work, but to have it in your home…"

"How does she deal with crime at work?"

"She's a criminal defense attorney. Erin Fitzgerald."

The officer sighed in recognition, and said, "I know who she is. She's the one with the red hair. Usually has it rolled up into a knot at the back of her head."

"That's her. I like to clip out the stories when she's in the newspaper. Show off my customer to the family. But to have something happen in your own house. That's different."

"We'll do our best to make it as easy for her as possible," he said. "The homicide detectives will be here any time now. We're taking the preliminaries, but they're the ones who will work the case. I hope they get here before she does."

As if on cue, they both turned when they heard Erin outside the door demanding to know what was happening. The second officer acting as sentinel said something they could not hear, but she responded in a severe authoritarian tone that she demanded he let her through.

The officer with Marguerite said, "Stay here." He looked as if he were going to help the other officer when they heard footsteps on the stairs and new voices. "The detectives are here."

Marguerite stepped inside when he left her. She saw Erin, at first aggressive and self-important, then watched when she collapsed in a chair. Marguerite knew they had told her what happened to her friend. Their association was not of friends or even close acquaintances, but she thought how alone she was in the world and how she needed a shoulder to lean on right now. Pushing past the officer, she went to Erin and put her arms around her. She felt a tension give way in Erin, and she knew she had been right. No one can be tough all the time.

The detectives steered the two women to the living room sofa. The first detective took charge of the interview, introduced himself as Detective Steve Macy.

"We need to process the whole apartment but I don't see any harm in you sitting here for now. It must be a great shock," giving his partner a guilty look as if realizing for the first time that she might have feelings. "It's not going to be possible for you to stay here tonight. Is there somewhere you can go?"

"Yeah. Yes, I have a place to go," Erin said. "I'll need to get a few things from the bedroom."

"You tell us what you need. We can't let you in there now. Besides, I don't think it would be a good idea, if you get my meaning."

Erin lost the rest of the color in her face. She understood his meaning.

"You'll want to ask me questions. I'd like to do that now and get it over."

Looking over at her, Marguerite thought how she was no longer the fierce litigator, but the victim of violence. Proving again how life can change in a moment.

"First. What's her full name?"

"Hermione Jones."

Marguerite and the detective frowned. Erin must have expected that reaction, because she spelled it and then said, "Her-my-oh-nee." She pulled out her cell phone, scrolled down, and read off Hermione's home address.

"We have a few questions to ask that will help us establish a timeline. When did you last speak with her?"

"That would be right after I went to see a client at the jail, around 1:00. She wanted to do a run, so we agreed that I would pick her up afterwards for late lunch," Erin said, glancing toward the patio door. Through the glass, she saw the drink glass sitting on the patio table and pointed it out to the detective. "It looks like she helped herself to a drink while she was waiting. There wasn't a lot else here."

"We saw that," he said. "The crime scene people will take the drink and the other contents away for testing. The medical examiner is almost positive the cause of death is poisoning, so they'll test anything she might have touched or consumed."

"Poison? Why would anyone want to hurt Hermione? I'm the only person she knows in Phoenix."

"It's a possibility that you were the intended target. This *is* your home. Have you received any recent threats? In your business, you must run into dissatisfied clients or folks that resent your representation of certain clients."

"I get my fair share of nasty letters, all of which would be in a file at the office. My paralegal collects them and keeps them in a file in case we have problems. I'll have her send them over."

"Is there anything about your friend that could be relevant? Boyfriends, problems at work?"

"I can't think of anything. She wasn't seeing anyone now, and she loved her work. I can't think of anyone that she ever mentioned that would want to hurt her."

"We'll have to consider both angles. Either someone wanted to kill you or her. Take my card. If you think of anything, call me. I don't have to tell you that the most insignificant fact can alter an investigation."

Once the paramedics arrived, he pointed to Erin. A young woman came to speak to both Erin and Marguerite. Having seen it on television, Marguerite understood why they came. It was not for the dead but for the living—to check for shock, or another condition brought on by the intrusion of a violent act in their lives. Once the young woman had looked them over, she gave them her cards to use if they needed to talk. That is when she asked Erin what she needed from the bedroom and retrieved a list of toiletries and clothing in a small suitcase.

Marguerite felt guilty thinking about the star treatment she was getting. She enjoyed the attention. Fantasizing herself as the center of attention later tonight, she had taken in all the activity by the police and the paramedics, regretting she had to leave and miss the crime scene people, but this would be in the papers and on the news.

Erin forced herself to stay alert against the exhausting emotion overtaking her until she could get out of there. A sense of horror came over her as she imagined the scene if she had been the one who walked in and found Hermione. Coming home, expecting the bright face of her friend to greet her, but instead finding her dead on the floor.

She had not experienced sudden death close up except through the dealings of her clients. She had scoured crime scene photographs detached and clinical as if the victims were not real but staged in those positions and surroundings for exhibition. She would never look at another violent death the same without knowing that every murdered man or woman left behind living victims. People who had to live with the knowledge that their loved one had died a miserable death. The tears were coming, but she forced them back until later, away from onlookers.

"Are you going to be okay?"

Erin looked startled. She had forgotten that Marguerite still stood next to her. "Oh, yes, I'll be fine. But what about you? You've had a great shock."

"I called my daughter. She'll have my whole family waiting for me at home. It's been upsetting but not like you. I didn't go down the hall, so I never saw her. Besides, I didn't know her."

"I guess it's a blessing you were spared that," Erin said. "I want to thank you for being there for me when I heard the news. I appreciate it." She reached into her purse and pulled two fifties from her wallet. "This is for you."

"I didn't earn that. I wouldn't feel right."

"Take it and don't argue. I know you count on this money." Erin pressed the bills into her hand and closed her fingers around them. "It's been a rough day for both of us."

Marguerite's muscular arms wrapped around Erin. Erin heard the older woman stifling her emotions. Marguerite pulled away, blinking back tears. "You're a kind woman. I will pray for you and your friend."

Erin watched Marguerite pick up her cleaning supplies and walk down to her car. Erin could not be sure if the wave of sadness came from knowing Hermione was dead or the fact that a kindhearted woman would turn down much needed money.

Once she had her bag, she turned over her home to the professionals photographing, processing, and searching. Her usual feelings about privacy had become irrelevant this afternoon to the point that she had no concern about anything they might see or misinterpret.

She knew they were watching her. She took one more look around the home she once thought she could never leave, and hurried down to her car where she could break down alone and unobserved.

CHAPTER SEVEN

When she had not been able to reach Tate by phone, Erin checked with Rachelle and learned he had two back-to-back emergency surgeries and would be unavailable until late. Erin took her chances and let herself into his place with a spare key he had loaned her when they met there for an out-of-town trip. She had forgotten about it until panic set in that she might have to go to a hotel. She thought about staying at his place as an alternative. Maybe he would say that she should have thought of him first, but after his ordeal with Henry, she did not know that the two of them commiserating together was the best choice.

After thinking through her predicament, she sent him a text that she had an emergency at her place and could not stay there. Was it okay to stay with him? She had smiled when she saw his response. Always a man to make words work hard, he had responded with one letter "k." She needed a laugh, and smiled thinking of the succinct and elegant letter that told her, *of course you can.*

Once inside the temporary sanctuary of Tate's condo, Erin dropped into the softness of his leather chair, tucked her feet under her, and wrapped her body in a throw. Instead of finding comfort in familiar surroundings, she had become disoriented and numb, lost in a surreal world, vulnerable and afraid, disconnected from the rest of life. Hermione had been an important person in her life, the anchor that kept her grounded. Without her, Erin felt exposed to a frightening unknown. In the worst part of this nightmare, she wondered if she were strong enough to cope without her. She shrugged off her morbid thoughts. What did Hermione always say? Self-pity was a dangerous road.

Erin jumped up, shook off the throw, and went to the kitchen to make a White Russian. She and Hermione drank those creamy cocktails when they were old enough to order them in a bar. She carried the drink, and her bag to the bedroom. She saw Tate's shirt, discarded and ready for the dry cleaners. On an impulse, she grabbed it, brought it to her face, and breathed in his earthy smells. His lingering scent created a soothing reminder of when their bodies locked together with only sweat between them. She pulled his shirt around her for comfort and tried not to cry.

Tate had a break between surgeries, and took time to read Erin's message again. He wondered what happened. Maybe a burst pipe or something else that made staying there impossible. Whatever the problem, he warmed knowing he would see her if he got out of here in time. He smiled imagining her falling into his bed, her long hair loose, draped across the pillows, the milky softness of her toned body nestled naked under his sheets, sniffing in his scent when her face touched down on his pillowcase. Her subtle eroticism welcomed him inside. Then, he was there in the room with her, listening to her soft snoring as he stripped down, anticipating the moments ahead when he slipped under the cover next to her, the excitement when his legs moved against hers, and she started to wake.

"Doctor, they're ready for you."

He jumped at the sound of the nurse's voice. Partly flustered, partly annoyed, he made a grudging move to follow her. By the time he scrubbed and prepared to start the procedure, thoughts of Erin had dissipated, lost to the immediacy of the patient's needs in front of him.

Erin woke up to the harsh reality that life went on. She had a pang of loneliness when she saw the empty space next to her that told her Tate had not been able to get away from the hospital again. She sank deeper into his king-sized bed, and studied the masculine tones surrounding her. This room comforted her more than the others did, maybe because he spent most of his time at home in here. His essence imprinted on every object, like the traces of cologne in his shirt that she slept in and in the sheets she hid under now.

She had told him once that his extravagant lifestyle, from his luxury condo with its lavish furnishings, to his Pagani sports car, was an affront to her Spartan sensibilities. This morning, she could not resist indulging in every aspect of his home's luxuriant comfort. She shook her head and laughed at how easy the trap she set for herself with that kind of thinking. At least she could find something amusing after what happened.

She wrapped his bulky robe around her, and went to the kitchen. This morning, the continuing masculine theme throughout the rest of the apartment grounded her and gave her a sense of protection. Not a fan of stainless steel, she found it had a comfortable home here in the large eat-in kitchen with a long pine table and chairs. She made coffee in his Chemex coffee pot and sat at the table to stare out of the window. Nothing much to see this high up, but the clouds moving by provided a sense of weather and time. She remembered that Hermione would never experience either again and started to cry.

As easy as it was to wallow in her grief, she had responsibilities to others that she could not ignore. She could not relegate interactions with clients to others in the office. One was Imogen. The other was a new client interview at eleven.

She had a piece of toast with her coffee and then showered. While she dressed, she started plotting her defense strategies for her current cases. The fatiguing labor of criminal law had always been her self-diagnosis for troubles. She had to focus on the needs of someone else and plan how she intended to help them. Murder, robberies, assaults, everything but rape, she had made her reputation getting them lighter sentences or proving them innocent. Like her hero, she spent long nights in the law library or talking with private detectives, using whatever means necessary. One thing she knew now was that she wanted to be on the other side of the aisle in the trial for the person who killed Hermione.

She blinked back tears to keep her make-up intact, the supreme feminine argument to fend off unwanted emotional outbursts. Still she applied more concealer under her eyes, grabbed her purse, and left the key on the console table by the door with a "thank you" note under it. Maybe that was not necessary, but she did not want him to think she took anything for granted.

When she arrived at the office, life in the pit went on as usual. Clattering keyboards, smells from printers and copy machines running, muffled sounds of telephone conversations. The partners were in their offices, some with clients or talking into their phones. She noticed a definite hush come over the room when she walked toward her office. They had heard what happened by now, and were watching her for cues on her mental state, not unlike she, Lorraine, and Barry had done with Tate the other night.

"Good morning, Ms. Fitzgerald. How are you holding up?" Penny Lykins handed her a mug of coffee on her way into her office.

"I'm doing as well as I can. I think the work will do me good. Take my mind off what happened. Any messages?"

"Yes. The Assistant District Attorney called. She said the DA's moving forward with the murder charge. Like you figured, he contends Imogen had present ability when she denied he was dead and had the present ability to conceal the murder. He agreed to hold off until the psychiatrist presents his findings."

Erin sighed. "At least that gives us more time. Anything else."

"Tim Actworth, the new client, called to say he might be fifteen minutes late."

"Let's take advantage of that. See what you can find out on the therapist's murder. Any background on her. I want to get an idea of her personal life, family, what men she saw, and what type of patients she had. You know the kind of stuff I mean."

"Right," Penny said, jotting notes on her notepad. "I've heard of her. She promoted herself as an intuitive therapist slash psychic slash scientist."

"Interesting," Erin said. "Sounds like a guarantee for immediate results. That's an angle to consider. Get what you can on her successes. And any dissatisfied clients, too."

"That should be easy. She made frequent appearances on the local talk show circuit."

"Finally, get that file of threatening letters over to the

police. They said that I might have been the target. If you can think of anyone that's not in the files, please pass it on. Detective Steve Macy is the detective in charge of that case. Give him whatever he asks for that is legally appropriate."

"I will," Penny said. "I just want to say how sorry I am about your friend. I don't know how you're coping."

"I'm lucky because I have you to keep me propped up," Erin said. She blinked wet eyes. "Now get to work, please. Oh, and if Tate calls, put him right through unless the client is here."

"Too late. The client's here."

Erin watched Penny seat Tim Actworth in the conference room. She saw him nod a dismissal to the offer of coffee, but Penny set out bottled water anyway. His type reminded her that being a lawyer for her was a calling, not a profession.

She smiled at those stereotypes that all lawyers made the big bucks. She had months when making her condo payment turned into a magician's juggling act. The truth was many of her clients could not afford to pay her standard rates. So many were career criminals, incapable or resistant to holding down a regular job, but others were lower income, uneducated individuals who got caught in the legal system's machinery. She made most of her money on her few high profile cases, or when things were tight, take a personal injury case where criminal negligence was involved.

Tim Actworth, a young man, had hired her to defend him for the murder of his therapist. According to him, the evidence was circumstantial and could fit any other of her patients. He said the police looked at him for it because he argued with her that morning. This was one for Perry Mason, she thought. Her childhood hero, the fictional criminal attorney created by Erle Stanley Gardner, an author who was an attorney himself inspired by his time in the justice system. That's who it would take to keep this boy from death row, but she had to try.

"Good morning, Mr. Actworth. Do you mind if I call you Tim?"

"No, ma'am."

His polite manner surprised Erin. "Let's jump right in. Describe to me the relationship you had with Delia Ferguson."

Well," Tim said. "We got along fine. I went to her because my girlfriend thought I needed help fitting in. She thought I'd be more successful. I guess I'm kind of shy around folks. I'm not from around here and feel out of place."

"I see. So Delia was helping you?"

"I guess, but I didn't like the way she kept suggesting all these changes. I told my ma about it, and she said I didn't need therapy. She said if folks didn't think I fit in here, I should come home where I was appreciated."

"Did you and Delia argue this point?"

Tim sniffed. "Not exactly what I would call arguing. When I told her what my ma said, Delia insulted her. I don't take that lying down, and I told her so. Then she started insulting me, telling me I didn't appreciate all she was doing for me. To be honest, I thought she must've been kind of off. I paid her for every visit. It's not like I'm a charity case."

"Of course not," Erin said. "That seems harsh coming from a professional. Then what happened?"

"I guess this happened the day somebody killed her. I decided to get out of there because she was getting so worked up. She had me so upset, I went out the wrong door and almost ran into her next patient."

"Did you notice this other patient?"

"Some woman. I didn't really look at her, because Delia was still yelling. I kept turning back to make sure she wasn't going to throw something at me."

"Sounds like a very heated exchange. What did you do when you left?"

"I had to cool off, so I drove around Phoenix, sightseeing like. I had to decide whether to go back home or stay here. The only reason to stay was Charlene, but she didn't seem to be happy with who I am. I figured I'd talk to her about what happened with Delia, and as my ma says, 'The truth shall set you free.'"

"And did it?"

Tim's expression darkened. "Yes it did. I realized Charlene was looking for someone to change into who she wanted, not interested in me as I am. I went to pack and would be home now if the police hadn't shown up wanting to question me."

Erin's empathetic nature took over. Another reason she would never be rich.

Tim raised his head to look her in the eye. "I don't have much money, but if you'll represent me, I promise I'll pay you every cent as soon as I'm home and working again. I brought three hundred with me."

"That'll be fine. We'll work out an arrangement. Give Penny the money on your way out and she'll write you a receipt for the retainer. This won't cause you a hardship, will it?"

"No ma'am. I have enough to live on for about two months. I hope this don't go on that long though. I'd like to get back home to my normal life as fast as I can."

Erin smiled. "From what you're telling me, the evidence they have against you can apply to any number of current and former patients. Give me a few days to review your case, and I'll get back to you with a plan."

"You don't know what a relief this is." He stood when he saw Erin rising from her chair. He extended his hand, and said, "Thank you, ma'am."

Erin watched him leave and wondered where back home was. She also wondered if all the men back home were as polite as Tim. Or did Tim's mother know how to raise a man?

In answer to the call by Penny Lykens, Detra Ferguson checked her mother's patient files that the police had allowed her to pack up for long-term storage. While she had the obligation to store the records the legal time limit, the patients could request copies of their files for their next therapist. She agreed to any request, but she told them she would take an inventory of every scrap of paper before releasing anything. Almost complete, the file inventory listed every patient from her mother's computer and cross-matched with electronic notes, schedule books and physical files. To her surprise, the murder suspect's file was present in each category. What she had not expected was to find another patient's physical file missing. She saw that patient, a female, twice a week for the last six months. She used the name of Polly, but with no last name.

Before returning Penny's call, Detra telephoned Detective Macy.

"I thought you should know," she said.

"What about electronic notes? Anything there?"

"I looked at those, and she made notes about her sessions with the woman. She explains the woman considered herself a public figure and was adamant about secrecy, so my mother must have known her real name. If

Polly stole her file, she must not have known about the electronic notes. I've saved everything I have on her and will send them to you. Without a name, I wouldn't know who to contact for permission. My mother kept her word about keeping her anonymous, but I hope to find even a notation before I finish."

"I appreciate you telling me about this. Whether she killed your mother or not, it's curious that she found the opportunity to get into the office to remove her file after your mother's death."

"That's what I thought. I want my mother's killer caught and punished, but I don't want a witch-hunt where the press crucifies the wrong person. We've all seen enough of that. You can never undo that kind of damage, even if you're not a celebrity. That goes against what my mother was about and would dishonor her memory."

Detective Macy hesitated. "We don't want a miscarriage of justice either. You can be sure we'll investigate this new angle. I guarantee you we'll get the right person."

Detra tried to speak but felt that absence of movement in her throat. After holding her breath for several seconds to stop the tears, she said, "Thank you," and disconnected the call. She could not keep her emotions stuffed down any more and started to cry.

"Whoever you are, you better hope the cops get you before I do."

CHAPTER EIGHT

Tate had an additional trauma surgery the night before that lasted almost eight hours. By ten thirty that morning, he finally had the opportunity to give into the exhaustion behind the closed door of his office. Every muscle ached, a physical exhaustion that threatened to affect his thinking if he did not rest soon. Maintaining mental acuity came from years of conditioning, but he had to rely on regular fitness and strength training to counter the physical toll on his body after hours on his feet. Once he checked on a few patients admitted in the hospital, he looked forward to his hot tub, a good meal, and sleep.

Rachelle knocked, and stuck her head around the door before he had a chance to answer." I don't know if you heard since you've been in surgery so long."

"Heard what?"

"I'm so sorry, after all you've been through, but I think you should know. I heard on the news last night that Erin's friend Hermione was murdered in Erin's apartment yesterday."

"What?" Tate grabbed his desk for support." That can't be right."

"I'm so sorry. It's horrible. I thought I should let you know so you're prepared. The police called for an appointment to ask you questions. You know, general questions about enemies or threats against Erin."

He looked at his cell phone and remembered Erin's message. Looking back through the words now, panic rippled deep in his gut. He had let her down by not being with her. He had only met Hermione once, but he knew how much that friendship meant to the both of them since grade school. Erin had once said they were part of each other's common history that she shared with no one else. Imagining losing someone like that, he likened that to losing his entire family and friends all at once—all the links to his own past gone.

"Can you find out where she is? I'll return the call to… what's the detective's name?"

"Steve Macy," Rachelle said. "I'll bring the number."

He made the call, but had to leave a message.

When Rachelle tracked Erin down at her office, Tate could not believe she went to work. Rachelle put the call through to his extension once Penny put Erin on the line.

"I just heard. I'm so sorry about Hermione. And I'm sorry I couldn't be there. How are you holding up? And *what* are you doing at the office?"

"Letting me stay at your place was support enough. If I'd had to stay at a hotel, I think I would've broken down I couldn't make sense of how you felt the other day until I indulged in serious self-pity for a few hours. I needed that time to be alone, just like you did. Now, I need to get on with my work, be around people who need my help. How can I be strong for my clients if I can't be strong for myself?"

"I'm leaving here soon. I'm beat. Come over when you're done there. We can talk about all of this then." He hesitated. "You stay at my place as long as you need to. No argument."

"Thank you."

He could tell by the shakiness in her voice that she was

more upset than she wanted to admit. Many people might not get it, but they were alike in that they both dealt best with emotional issues by the healing power of hard work. She had to take care of the clients more for her than for them.

"Any news on Imogen? Anything you can tell me, of course," he said.

"The judge ordered a psychiatric evaluation. They transferred her to Forensic Services Division for the Correctional Health Services Restoration to Competency program this afternoon. From my meetings with her in jail, I believe that's the best treatment. I'm sorry the news is grim. If she weren't so scattered and I could get straight answers from her, I'd feel better. All she wants to talk about is helping her friend who she can't remember."

"I haven't figured out how I feel about any of this yet. It's like a bad dream. I can't begin to imagine what this will do to their children." He paused when he realized his selfishness in turning this around and making this about him instead of her. "When are you leaving the office?"

"I've had my meeting with the new client already. I have notes to type and a few phone calls. I'll be out of here in about an hour."

"I'll see you at my place, then. Doctor's orders."

She laughed. "I wondered when you were going to get around to using that corny line." She laughed. "A quiet evening sounds lovely."

"See you there." He disconnected the call and leaned back. Two deaths of close friends within days of the other had to be the worst thing that could happen to two people in a young relationship. He rubbed his forehead. *What next?*

He checked his mail for anything pressing. In the black mesh basket on his desk, he pulled and sorted envelopes according to size. One small beige packet looked like an invitation. He slid the metal letter opener through its top, and pulled out the small card. Happy anxiety for the distraction, he started to read the typed note. His momentary diversion turned to irritation when he read,

Derren,

We want to thank you for the opportunity to meet with you to discuss our mutually beneficial marketing plan. To thank you for your valuable time, please accept the enclosed theatre tickets.

Regards. Ben.

Tate checked the outside of the envelope. His firm's name, but with Derren's name as principal. He fought the instinct to track him down for a confrontation. He was too tired. He would take care of the situation when he was better prepared. Erin needed his comfort and support right now, not more problems.

He tossed, shredded, or set aside for filing the rest of the mail. He looked down at his trembling hands. He sat back and took a deep breath. This was getting him nowhere.

"Rachelle, I'm leaving now. I'm still on call, but I'll be reachable by text if you need me."

"Tell Erin I'm sorry," Rachelle said.

"I'll do that. See you tomorrow."

When he walked in, he saw Erin leaning back on the sofa, waiting for him with wine glasses and a bottle of their favorite French burgundy. She stood up as he reached her and leaned in to put his arms around her. She buried her face in the folds of his jacket, her hair loose, sweaty strands dangling down the sides of her face. He smoothed her hair and kissed the top of her head. She leaned into him and her body relaxed.

"I'm so glad to see you," she said, clinging to keep him from letting go.

"I liked Hermione. She didn't deserve that."

She pulled back, and looked up at him with something he had not seen in her before. Was that fear? "I still can't come to terms with this. Who could hate me that much to want to kill me? All I've done to help my clients, I find it impossible to think any of them would hate me. God knows, I don't have many close friends—I work too much for socializing. I can't imagine the few friends I have developing a hatred of me to want to kill me. It's not real."

"Like Imogen and Henry," he said.

"I know you're suffering, but I still want you to comfort me. Selfish, huh? I guess if there's any solace, it's that I didn't find Hermione's body. When I saw how Marguerite handled herself, I don't know how she coped so well."

He poured the wine as he listened. When she paused, he looked up and said, "I don't know about you, but I can't relive those moments again. Just when you think you're okay the visual comes back, and you feel worse than when it first happened. I want to remember Henry and Imogen as they were."

"You're right. I have a lifetime of memories with Hermione to keep me company." Erin sipped her wine, leaned back, and looked out at the late evening sky. He wondered how long she would hold back the tears. The strain in her face said not too long. He needed to distract her.

"I planned to tell you something later, but now is a

good time for you to put on your lawyer hat." He leaned back on the sofa arm to watch her while she slipped off her shoes and drew her legs up to rest across his lap.

"Go on," she said. She picked up her wine glass and poised it under her lips.

"Don't say, I told you so."

"Promise." She smiled. "Go on, I'm intrigued."

"Derren is up to something. Rachelle routed a letter to me by accident. Or maybe on purpose. Seems he's preparing to make *marketing* decisions that smell like kickbacks. I don't know the details yet. We're mainly a cash business, but Derren receives a good portion of his patient fees from federal healthcare programs. That makes this issue more complicated."

"How do you want to handle it?"

"I decided not to beat his face in. He'd end up as one of my trauma patients, and I'd have to patch him up." He laughed. "Mostly joking. But I gave this some serious thought. I'm not doing anything. He could say what he did was research for both of us. Fact gathering before he talked to me. That would put me on the defensive. Instead, I'll keep an eye on him to see how far he'll go. When I have something concrete, I'll approach him."

"Gathering evidence. I think I've made an impression on you. It's a strategy that puts you in control."

"That's what I think. Suspicion is a slow-acting poison in any type of relationship."

"Good analogy," Erin said. "That's how it happens with my clients, whether we're talking about a personal relationship or issues between business associates."

"It's not a pleasant feeling suspecting someone might be getting ready to stab you in the back. The hard part is pretending I'm not angry."

"That won't be too difficult. You can be a mask of

cool reserve when you want."

Tate laughed, but felt his face redden at that intimate observation. "You're getting to know me well."

CHAPTER NINE

Tate arrived at the office looking forward to the surgery-free day, and easy appointments for Botox, Juvederm fillers, and follow-ups. He checked the day's schedule, and saw he had a new patient consult, then consecutive appointments with Monica Aames, Devon Bateman, Fleur Sanders, and Frankie Campbell. This is the first time seeing Imogen's friends since *it* happened. The idea of answering questions about the details made him anxious, but he had to get through it as best he could.

His first appointment, Clara Beal, had asked for a consultation for a labiaplasty. He guessed she was around fifty, looked like she took care of herself, but showed obvious signs of many poorly executed procedures. It was not unusual that a new patient came to him to correct another doctor's work, or because her previous plastic surgeon refused to do a particular procedure.

Clara listened, but asked no questions. He thought she did not intend to until she looked him in the eye and said, "What guarantee do I have that the vaginoplasty won't fail if I have sex with a man with a very large *part*, if you get my drift?"

He pressed his lips together. He had mastered the skill of expressionless reaction, so that all an observant person might detect was the involuntary twitch of his lower lip.

"That won't happen if the procedure is performed

correctly, but you can have this discussion with the doctor who will perform that procedure. This consultation is for the labiaplasty only."

"Oh, I thought that was all taken care of together. It's a relief to know, anyway. Not that I have a particular man in mind, but hope springs eternal. My divorce is almost final." She winked, and scooted down to the table. "So, are you going to examine me or what?"

When he left Clara's examining room, he relaxed when he read Monica's name on the file hanging outside the next room. He looked forward to talking to a familiar face.

"Hey, Monica," he said as he walked in.

"You poor man," Monica said. "How are you holding up? What a horrible thing to have happen."

"I'm doing fine." His face reddened, and his facial muscles relaxed from the smile he had worn seconds before. The forced expression gave him an unemotional stiffness he did not like. He should have prepared for this. Monica and Imogen are friends.

"If I had suspected, I would've gone into her house after the fundraiser. Thinking back, I might have known deep down something wasn't right, but I ignored my instincts because I wanted to get back to the reception."

"I don't think anyone would have been able to guess. It's not the kind of thing you expect to happen with your friends."

Monica shook her head. "I miss Imogen already. I feel a big void without her. It's so sad."

Not wanting to encourage her to keep talking, he left the room for supplies that he knew were already in the cabinet. He returned with a small bottle and a syringe, and placed the small ice packs on her forehead.

After an awkward silence, she said, "Botox touch-up

today."

"So, it's been three months already," he said, looking in her file.

"I think it's only been two months, but I'm going to Chapala again and want to look my best."

"When are you leaving?"

"On Sunday, if all goes well. Of all the luck, Troy has a friend with a Cessna Latitude eight-seater plane who invited me along."

"Lucky you," he said. "Feel numb yet?"

"Yes. I decided since work was slow, I should enjoy myself somewhere cheap. And spend time with Troy and our friends, too, of course. You can't beat free transportation in a spanking new private plane."

"Of course not," he said. He tossed the ice packs onto a tray on the counter and filled the syringe with the Botox Cosmetic. "Close your eyes and frown," he said. After she relaxed the frown, he began the tedious job of injecting the Botox under her skin into the muscle tissue beneath. When he finished, he reminded her she had to stay prone for fifteen minutes to prevent the serum from moving down with gravity and left the room. As he shut the door, he glanced back and saw Monica's questioning look that he pretended not to see.

Her surprise was justified. His habit was to stay to keep her company, but today he was not up for reliving the nightmare of how he found Henry, how he felt about finding his dead body, and what he thought will happen to Imogen. He passed the reception area on the way to his office and saw Devon and Fleur waiting. He shuddered. More of the same.

Before he reached his office, Rachelle hurried over toward him. "Excuse me, Doctor, but Frankie Campbell asked if you had time to give her a longer appointment so she can talk to you about more surgery. I thought that if we put Devon and Fleur in rooms at the same time that would give you a little extra time for her. Dr. Davide doesn't have patients this afternoon."

"That sounds okay. Call me when they're ready. Oh, give them both ice packs, too," he said. He thought that might dilute his time alone with them to avoid chatting opportunity. But he started to have second thoughts once he reached his office. He stared out at the desert plants blocking his view. He did not feel good about being abrupt with Monica. This was not like him. He initiated those friendly chats with his long-term patients as much as they did. A dynamic group of women, all of them could charm the pants off any man, but the exchange was playful and friendly more than sexual. A refreshing disparity to the Clara Beals of the world. He got up and returned to her room.

"You're about done. How are you doing?"

She looked relieved. "Great. Just resting and dreaming of Mexico. A busy day?"

"Yes, as a matter of fact, two of your cohorts are in the lobby and another due soon. Ganging up on me today?"

"That's our plan, except we'll nab you in the parking garage when you least expect it."

"I'll carry my feather tickler. Make all of you laugh so hard, you'll form new wrinkles."

"That's sounds lethal. We might have to reconsider our plan."

He motioned for her to get up, and checked her forehead once more.

"I'm glad you're okay. Really," she said. She gave him a hug, and made her way toward the door.

"Have a good time in Mexico," he said.

With Rachelle busy on the phone with a patient, Tate led Fleur and Devon to adjoining examining rooms. They giggled about sharing the appointment.

"Ooh, Fleur. Tate's *rooming* us together!"

Fleur could be a devil when she thought about it, so he was ready when she said, "Wow. So this is what a threesome with you is like? First you room her, then you room me. I'm glad to see you're up to keeping both of us happy at the same time."

"And what man wouldn't with the two of you?" he said.

From the next room, he heard Devon say, "What's going on over there? I'm getting jealous."

"Wait your turn, Chicky," Fleur said. "You'll get him when I'm finished."

"Every man's dream is to be fought over by beautiful women."

They both had Botox, giving him a break from the more intensive fillers. He kept their individual time limited but still had enough conversation time for the happy medium he needed. Between Fleur's dirty jokes and Devon's sly comments, the last few days seemed distant. He was sorry to see them leave. They played off each other like a comedy act—a refreshing non-competitiveness he did not see too often in women.

In contrast, Frankie wore a serious frown, maybe because of her ambitious nature and the pressure to run a business on her own. He had grown nervous around her more than once in the examining room. The uncomfortable feeling, unlike Clara Beal's obvious flirtations, came from a disconcerting undercurrent he could not define. Last week, she came in to ask about a facelift that she did not need. Today, she wanted to discuss details of a necklift. For all her swagger, she had approached him with a respectful deference, but lately she seemed present only behind a veil. Her presence had lost something significant, and if she had not been one of his long-timers, he might have discouraged more appointments. On the other hand, a good paying cash client was not something to turn away.

"Hi, Frankie." He sat on the wheeled stool across from her.

"I decided to ask you about a necklift. Maybe I don't need the facelift, but more of a tightening around the neck. How do you do that?"

Tate pulled out a sketch sheet from her file and pulled out a pencil from the depth of his lab coat. He let out a loud sigh and rolled the seat closer to her so she could watch him sketch.

"Similar to the pre-op for a facelift, I'll mark your face, neck, and jawline while you're standing and before you're anesthetized. Once you're on the table, we'll apply an antiseptic to make sure the skin surface is sterile. I'll make an incision just under your chin wide enough to expose the platysma muscle. Depending on the volume of fat, which in your case is minimal, I would sculpt around the jawline and cut out any fat underneath the platysma muscle. Any questions so far?"

He looked over, but Frankie's eyes never left the paper. "No, go on. Please."

"To tighten the neck, I'll suture the muscle back together with a curved needle, in about four stitches from side to side from the base to underneath the chin, much like corseting the area. Then, I'll suture that area. The next step is to tighten the skin along the jawline up the ear. I will have marked you already for the incision around the ears. After re-draping and repositioning the skin, I will cut off the excess at the marking around the ear without interfering with the natural hairline."

"That sounds painful."

"You'd be unconscious during the procedure," he grimaced. "When you wake up, you'll be wearing a compression garment or neck binder that you'll continue to wear for the first few weeks. With that and pain medication, you won't feel as bad as you imagine."

Why is she wasting my time? He was positive now, but what could be her motive. Maybe she was gathering information for someone else.

"Well, I have some thinking to do about it. Whether I want to do it and if I believe that I do or don't need it yet," she said.

"I think that's a good idea, Frankie. Aging is a normal function of the body. It's important to keep in mind that while the surgery gives the appearance that age has reversed, aging continues to happen afterward in much the same manner it did before. What you're seeing now will inevitably start to occur again. Waiting for five years will give you a significant benefit, whereas having the surgery now will have less benefit and will have a declining benefit in the same five years."

"How depressing," Frankie said.

"Improving someone's appearance is what I do, but I want you to be informed about your options. I'd rather you wait than to spend money on procedures that won't make you happy in the long term."

"I appreciate that."

"If you want to discuss it further, make another appointment. We can talk about other non-surgical options, if you still believe you want to do something." He stood and reached out to shake her hand to signal the end of the visit.

"Thanks, Dr. Tate. I appreciate your time." She started

to follow him out to the reception area, but half way down the corridor, she gasped. "Oh, I forgot my compact. I'll be right back."

He spent a few minutes to give instructions to Rachelle. His concentration and acuity kicked in again, and his thoughts had moved on to the next patient.

Rachelle looked down the hallway. "Where'd she go?"

"She said she left a compact in the room, whatever that is. She should be right out."

But Frankie did not return. He and Rachelle exchanged curious looks. He walked back toward his office. He pushed the door open to find Frankie at his desk peering into one of his drawers.

"What are you doing?"

"Oh, Tate. I didn't want to bother you again. I thought I'd pop in and pick up literature on a facelift to take with me."

"You need to see Rachelle for those materials. The doctors' offices are off-limits to patients, no matter who they are."

"I'm so sorry. It won't happen again."

"I'm sure of that," Tate said.

She backed out of the room and scurried down the hall. He heard the door close. She had not stopped to ask Rachelle anything. The literature was an excuse. *She wanted to find something, but what the hell was she looking for in my office?*

CHAPTER TEN

With several murder cases on his desk, Detective Macy developed the habit of viewing all his cases every morning to keep his perspective fresh, as well as keep the known facts of each case at the front of his mind. His present caseload consisted of the Hermione Jones murder. Then the female medical student Jenny Marcus, found dead in the Sky Harbor parking garage, and the psychic therapist Delia Ferguson, found murdered in her office. He also kept the file on the Henry Vine murder on his desk, even if he knew the killer. He did not like the proximity to the Hermione Jones case. Too many overlapping characters, even if most were not suspects.

Another reason the Vine murder case stayed open owed to the instability of the prime suspect, his wife Imogen, who had trouble knowing if the sun was out much less the details of the murder. Her attorney, probably the actual target in the Jones case, took the position that until Imogen remembered she committed the murder, she would not advise her to confess only on an assumption that she did it.

The doctor who discovered the body gave a statement that she explained why she did it, but until she provided a lucid confession, they had to keep options open. Farfetched as it sounded, she could be covering up for someone else who killed her husband, and then snapped at the horror of what happened. You could never assume anything with people. It would do no harm to interview her friends to get her background.

Then there was the therapist. Her murder was not as clear-cut as they had thought in the beginning. Macy and his partner, Stokes, had believed they found Delia Ferguson's killer, a young man named Tim Actworth. They had spent time actively gathering supporting evidence when the victim's daughter discovered another suspect, a missing file for a different patient who had no connection to their prime suspect. Expecting to wrap that one up, now he had to start over by finding the mysterious patient, Polly. It could be they were right about Actworth, but as Detra had said, they had to be sure. That Fitzgerald woman was representing him too, which lead him to another new case.

Hermione Jones, a close friend of Erin Fitzgerald, murdered in Erin's apartment two days ago. They suspected poisoning. They had sufficient preliminary results that the poison had been introduced inside the water bottles. Erin did not recognize them as items she purchased. He would have to wait to find out the specific poison, but he was ready to start the search for strangers in the area or someone with a personal grudge against Erin. They would be walking on eggshells with this one. Erin Fitzgerald was tough enough when she defended her clients. He had no doubt she would be relentless until they found the murderer of her best friend.

His last open case was Jenny Marcus. He knew it was wrong, but he found the death of beautiful, intelligent young women, like her and Hermione Jones, more of a tragic loss. Owing to political correctness, he kept that opinion to himself, of course. With brains, looks, and ambition, Jenny Marcus had been destined to go places. If allowed to live out her life, her future would have been limitless to what she could have accomplished. From what her best friend had told him, she had a boyfriend, a doctor who her friend had suspected was married. "Otherwise, why the secrecy?" she had asked. He had to agree.

They had placed calls to her various professors to find out if she had a male mentor or a doctor who might have taken an interest in her. They either knew nothing or did not want to get involved. Since she was in her first year, she had been taking most of the required coursework, which meant lots of studying. Anyone or anything important enough in her life to detract her from her goal should become apparent. So far, that assumption had not proven itself.

As he saw it, all of these cases were unusual in that they involved upper middle-class individuals who did not live the high-risk lifestyle of his usual murder victims. Considering most murders that came across his desk stemmed from street crime or domestic disputes, he had his work cut out for him in delving into the lives of these victims to find out what made them deserving of murder.

He shook his head and sighed realizing that he had not one, but four high-profile cases. Not one drug addict or gang member in the bunch. He and his partner would need to be circumspect during the interviews with friends and family. Not so much for discretion, as most would assume, but to look underneath the public faces for motives without them figuring out what he was doing.

He decided to work two cases at once and interview the friends of Henry and Imogen Vine, who happened to be many of the same friends of Dr. Marsdon, who found his body. His romantic interest, Erin Fitzgerald, who was Imogen Vine's attorney, was tied to the Hermione Jones murder. He had no doubt that Erin was the target, and her friend's murder had been a mistake. They might be unrelated, but looking at mutual friends might reveal something otherwise missed.

Tate sat at his desk after the last appointment of the day to review the latest financial reports back from the accountant's office. This mundane task gave him a sense of normality that he needed. Most months he looked at the bottom line, saw a healthy profit, and filed the folder away. In addition to the need to ground himself, he wanted to check on the profitability of having a partner.

His motivation to bring in Derren had been cost sharing. With business booming, he had no problem making it on his own, but the ability to save more every month appealed to him for what might be the inevitable rainy day or early retirement in a changing political environment. It was easy to spend too much when you made significant income and then find yourself short later. He had no intention on allowing that to happen to him.

He reached for the office telephone, pressed the intercom button. "Rachelle, can you come in here?"

"I'll be right there."

He wondered how she stayed so perky all the time when she opened the door and smiled a questioning look.

"I need to see the travel and meals receipts for last month."

"Okay, be right back." She turned from the open door back to the depths of the office.

For the first time today, the office had a stillness, a tomblike atmosphere. Without the patients or Derren around, the modern office was cold and impersonal in spite of the warm tones of the interior surfaces and furnishings. He shrugged off a sudden chill. Rachelle returned with a fat manila folder and placed it in front of him.

"I'll return it later. I have to look for something."

"You're the boss."

"I'm not so sure about that. I think you're the real boss around here."

She smiled and left. He stared after her for a moment, trying to remember something.

Travel and meals expenses were heavier than usual in the financial statement compared to previous months. For him, luck would be a fine thing if he had the opportunity to go somewhere or to spend time eating at restaurants other than the occasional business lunch. The past month showed expenses higher than they had been the preceding month and the entire prior fiscal year. He hoped he could blame it on an accounting error.

The first paper he saw when he opened the file showed receipts for an expense report from Derren listing hotels, rental cars, and airfares. He saw various receipts stapled to the back of the report with notations of patient names or business contacts, none of which he recognized as specific to the practice. Their partnership agreement stated that personal expenses would be applied to the specific partner's drawing account rather than as a company expense. Before he said anything though, he had better make sure of his facts. But his gut told him he was right.

He had not experienced that festering sense of the betrayal since high school when he found out his girlfriend had cheated on him. Back then, his rage and indignation fueled the loss of trust and faith he had in her. After years of focus on his education, he had arrived at a time in his life where he thought those feelings were behind him. All it took was one look at these receipts, and he was eighteen again and gutted from realizing he still could be fooled.

He made copies of the receipts on his private scanner, and noted the names and nature of meal or trip. Looking up the individuals should be easy, and a quick call to verify the purpose of the meeting would either ease his mind or reinforce his growing suspicions. He noticed it was after five and thought the best thing was to use the scanned receipts and call from home in the morning.

He pressed the intercom button again, and called Rachelle to come back.

"You can put the file back. I'm done with it. And, um, don't mention I looked at this to *anyone*."

"Sure, no problem," Rachelle said, still smiling as she reached for the folder.

On his way out, he stopped at the front desk. Rachelle typed something into the computer and looked up with a question.

"Did those uniforms come in?"

"Yes, I'm wearing one of them." She stood up and spun around to show off a black one-button jacket and pencil skirt. "The others picked theirs up already."

"How do you feel not wearing your own clothes?"

"I thought I might not like it, but it's easy to get ready in the morning when you have a different outfit for every day of the week lined up for you. I love it. And when all the other girls are here and we have on the same clothes, I think of those exclusive spas. Very chic."

"No resistance, then?"

"Not when they saw the clothes and I told them the supplier outfits the employees for that big spa at the Biltmore," she said. "Great idea of yours."

"I can't take credit. My mother suggested it when my folks came during the summer."

"I love the concept. Just another reason I enjoy working here. My Alan said the other day what a better choice I made when I chose you over the podiatrist's office."

Tate laughed. "What was the deciding factor?"

"You paid more," Rachelle winked, stood up, and returned the folder to the cabinet. She hesitated, seemed to study something, and then looked back at Tate.

"I think you're a nice man to work for, so I'm going to tell you that I think your suspicions are right." She pointed a finger at Derren's closed office door. "Dr. Davide's been acting funny, secretive like, when he's at the front desk. Last week, he took a page of checks from the office account but never wrote in what they were for. When I asked him about them, he said he'd do it later. Until now, I wasn't sure if I should say anything."

"Thank you, Rachelle." Tate returned to his office, reached into his top drawer, and brought out a large envelope. He pulled out a card and went back to the front desk.

"A hundred dollar gift card?" Rachelle said when he handed it to her.

"You and Alan go out to a nice restaurant on me. Look at it as a bonus."

"Wow, this is great. Thank you."

"You've earned it," he said. "It's nice to know you've got my back."

A half hour later, he sat in his car, ready to start the engine. He did not like how he felt. There were too many bad things happening at once. He wondered if he had failed to notice important clues about Henry, Imogen, and Derren, by being too wrapped up his work.

Tate picked up two ready-to-go prime rib dinners from AJ's Market and headed home where he expected to find Erin. He had shrugged off those ancient insecurities by the time he arrived home. The return of his optimistic disposition put him back in control of his environment. He was not a helpless victim who allowed others to control his fate. Tomorrow, he would check out the receipts and, if necessary, call his lawyer regarding his options.

The elevator filled with the aroma of the hot meat steaming out of the bag. He looked forward to coming home. She was waiting for him. He could not remember when he last felt like that about someone. Not that he was ready for marriage, but he had a comfort knowing he had not worked so hard that he lost the ability to experience those human emotions. As much as he felt for Erin, she might not be the one, but now he knew there would be someone someday.

When he first crossed the threshold, he had a rush of disappointment that she had not come until he saw her on the balcony, immersed in the gurgling hot tub sipping wine. He set the food on the counter and slid open the glass door to the patio. The crispness of the winter air stung his skin. She turned when she heard him and looked up, smiling.

"Hi, there," she said.

"I'm surprised you're not cold out here. I've got some weight on you, and I feel the chill."

She started giggling. "Not yet."

"What?"

"You don't have any weight on me yet."

He liked seeing her laugh in that coquettish way she

did when half-sloshed on wine. He stood, watching the water surging up and down around her breasts.

"Seriously, I needed to think, and the cold helps me concentrate. Besides, the warm water wraps around me like a blanket. Are you coming inside? The water, that is."

Watching the outline of her naked body under the distortions of the foaming water, the naughtiness in her voice tempted him to strip down and dive in. Instead he laughed. "I brought food—prime rib. We both need to eat. The hot tub's not going anywhere."

"Food should be perfect about now," she said. "I've had three glasses of wine and no lunch." She stood straight up with amazing dexterity, wine glass in hand. Tate watched the water run down her exposed body and considered changing his mind. He reached down to pick up his robe and wrapped it around her as he helped her onto the rug and into his slippers. He grinned at the shameless way she wore his clothes, even when she had her own available.

By the time they set the table and filled their plates, Tate had poured a glass of red wine for him and refilled hers. They ate in silence for the first few minutes until Erin broke the silence.

"Imogen has her first appointment with the psychiatrist tomorrow. I'll go over to see her briefly. I wish she would snap out of her fog so I could get a better read on her."

"I'm still having a difficult time about her. She killed Henry, no matter what her state of mind. I guess they'll be able to tell if she's faking insanity?"

"They've seen it all. I don't think she has the background to know how to get away with it, but that's an opinion. I don't know her as well as you. By the way, their kids came into town to arrange for Henry's funeral.

They're shook up, as you would expect. They told me they're taking his body back to their hometown for a small service and burial, but no service here. I can see how they might see it that way."

"That will be a disappointment to a lot of people. I wonder if we should leave it or if I should ask the pastor at their church about a small service. I'll talk to the Judge tomorrow."

"That would be good. Not everyone has so many friends and acquaintances, so to not allow them to say goodbye is sad."

"Anything on your new case yet?"

"I think the case against my client will be dropped. Another patient has become known that looks better as a suspect. I have a question. Can a patient give a phony name to a doctor? Isn't there some checking required?"

"The therapist probably knew her real name but kept the notes in the alias for privacy reasons. If she worked on a cash basis that did not involve insurance, the patient could have given a phony name, and the therapist didn't ask questions. That's not the way we operate in my practice," he said. "Even if they pay in cash, we ask to see a driver's license for identification."

"So, unless there's a picture or the therapy notes documented under her real name, the cops might never find her."

"That's right," he said, and then added. "How are you holding up about Hermione?"

She winced. "I'm keeping it together. Work is a good distraction. What can I do about it anyway? If I could do something to bring her back, I would do what it takes. The worst part is I have to deal with the fact that my best friend since childhood most likely died in my place. There's no pill or therapy that will change that, even after the police find this person." Her voice faded to a whisper.

Tate reached over and took her hand.

She took a deep breath. "It's thinking about the things you wished you'd said, or the places you wish you could share one more time. What decisions you'd make if you knew your time was limited. That's the worst of it."

"You're right. I think about that with Henry. He teased me that I had worked so hard all my life that I hadn't learned to have fun. He would joke about insuring my surgeon's hands for a million dollars then send me mountain climbing on Mount Everest." He liked that one. "All kidding aside, he took a fatherly interest in me and wanted me to learn to lighten up and enjoy my success."

"Did you ever learn to do that?"

"No way. I'm going to work until I go blind or senile, then I'll think about having fun."

"Work is your fun. No one could be the workhorse you are if it wasn't."

"Right again. It's not easy for people to understand that I'm not a nine-to-fiver. I'm glad you do. It makes my life easier."

"I understand it because I'm like that, too," she said and drained her glass.

He went for the bottle to refill both their glasses, and paused to stare out the window. He found an unexpected calm between them that he would not have thought possible after the last couple of days. But at the edge of his consciousness, he sensed a brewing storm set aside for tomorrow. He turned on the gas fireplace, and settled in next to her again to watch the glow of the flames play on the highlights of her hair.

"Any suspects in your case?" Tate leaned in to take a strand of her long hair between his fingers. Its smooth texture brushed against the back of his hand like a tickler.

"No, I can't think of anyone. Lawyers are supposed to have enemies around every corner, but I represented innocent people who were acquitted. No one outside the case would have been angry about that. Granted, I've known people who've lashed out at attorneys through their grief because the punishment minimized the value of their friend or relative, but that's not me. I haven't defended hardened criminals and serial killers who I've helped to put back on the street. Imogen is the first client I've had who *confessed*, but why would anyone want to keep me from defending her?"

"Imogen couldn't have anything to do with this. Maybe this has nothing to do with your work. Someone from your personal life?"

"Until we started seeing each other, I hadn't had much of a private life, although that doesn't preclude me having one. Most of my friends are from college and law school who have moved on with their own careers in other cities. Some are colleagues here in Arizona that I socialize with occasionally."

"I meant more in the line of men, like a stalker. Have you received any creepy valentines or mysterious bouquets?"

"Sorry. As far as I know, I haven't met anyone like that, knock on wood." She rapped lightly on his forehead with her knuckles "You know me—an old-fashioned working girl keeping her head down against the storm."

"Old-fashioned working girl, huh." He did not bother to hold back a laugh.

CHAPTER ELEVEN

Imogen sat on the edge of the chaise, leaning sideways against the raised backrest. *So, this is a shrink's office? Not as vulgar as I expected.* The doctor in his white coat, stood with his back to her as he wrote something in a file, probably her file. Why she had to be here at all was a mystery to her. She told them she killed Henry. What else did they want from her?

He turned around and looked at her for a moment before speaking. "Mrs. Vine, I'm Dr. Davenport. May I call you Imogen?"

"Fine."

"Are you comfortable? If not, you can sit somewhere else."

Imogen looked at a stiff, commercial office chair, looked at the chaise longue. "Do I have to lie down?"

"No. Make yourself comfortable."

Imogen moved to the other seat, taking on a fixed, relaxed posture.

"Better?"

"Yes," Imogen said. She watched him take a seat opposite her, and set his pad and pen on his lap.

"I've received your preliminary information, your health history, family background, and medications. I understand you've been through a lot this past year. Do you feel comfortable talking about the cancer?"

"Sure," Imogen said. "I never dreamed I would get

breast cancer. I think I believed I was invincible, like cancer was that thing that only happened to other people. I watched the marathon runners, listened to their stories not thinking those stories would ever have relevance for me. I felt so removed from them, only touched by the passing pity for the unfortunates in the world. When the diagnosis sank in that I was vulnerable like everyone else, I still couldn't make it real. I knew my life was finished. I said as much to Henry, that we lost our Camelot."

"Tell me about that time. How did you discover you had a problem? Close your eyes. Put yourself back in time. What was going on in your life?"

Imogen thought what a soothing voice he had, almost hypnotic. Contrary to the anxiety she expected, she relaxed and found recalling that time gave her inner peace.

Session One

Devon's Rottweiler, Roman, raised his one hundred thirty pound frame, rested his paws on Imogen's breasts, and pushed her backward onto the console table at the front door.

"Oh, for crying out loud, Devon. Can't you control that dog," Imogen said. She grasped Roman's paws and pushed him down to the floor.

"I'm sorry. I've never seen him jump on anyone before. Roman, go to bed," Devon said, pointing an authoritarian finger toward the end of the living room.

"Are you okay, Imogen?"

They watched Roman, head down, walk toward his oversize dog bed. "I'll live. I'm just glad I'm not wearing anything expensive. What's come over that dog, anyway? He usually walks up to me and sits with that slobbery tennis ball in his mouth, and waits for me to play."

"Beats me. I'll keep an eye on him to make sure he doesn't do that again. With his size, he could kill a person. I hope he's not going rabid. Good thing you were next to the table. Otherwise, you'd have been flat on your back. Are you sure you're okay? You're sure he didn't hurt you?"

"My bra isn't feeling too comfortable right now, but I guess it's normal to have bruising with an impact like that. I'll be fine. Don't worry."

When Imogen opened her eyes, Dr. Davenport was watching her. His soft brown eyes exuded sympathy and kindness, the quality of putting others at ease. For a few moments, lost in the past, she thought how easy to pretend the last few days were part of a nightmare, not the ugly reality.

"This afternoon, let's continue where we left off," Davenport said, smiling.

"I think I'd like that," Imogen stood and reached out to shake his hand.

Devon's shaky hands pressed on her left breast. She closed her eyes while she slid her fingers across the area over and around the lump. She was amazed at how quickly the lump had formed, but more afraid of what it meant. All those months supporting Imogen, she had not once imagined this could happen to her. After all, she was only thirty-six, in good health, and no history of any kind of cancer in her family. Knowing the responsible action was to call her doctor for an urgent appointment, she could not find the courage to pick up the phone.

She visualized her future—a damaged body from

extreme chemotherapy, loss of hair, and months of recuperation. Devon did not know if she could make it with the same dignity as Imogen had shown. Throughout her ordeal, she had heard other women around Imogen complain that the treatment was as difficult, or worse, than the disease. No doubt an exaggeration, but the comments had frightened her to the extent she did not want to find out.

She could not take her eyes away from the mirror. She took an objective assessment of her body. Smooth, tight, toned, little sun damage and great skin texture. Of all those attributes, she admired her round, firm breasts the most. Long in the tooth by some standards, she had feigned off the pudginess of other women her age by working out regularly, eating right, and allowing herself to indulge in a good drunk not more than once a month. She ran her hands over both breasts as a gesture to help her remember. There might be a day when they would be gone, replaced with emptiness and a deep angry scar.

She turned away from the mirror, wrapped herself in a bulky robe, and fell into her bedside chair. One part of her wanted to deny what she needed to do, while the other part knew she had to make the call to the doctor's office. To avoid calling her doctor bordered on insanity. She had too many plans for her life for it to end now. She reached for her cell phone, scrolled down, and pressed a number.

Once Monica answered, Devon said, "I found a lump in my breast. Will you go with me to the doctor? I can't face this alone."

"Devon, of course I'll go with you. When did you notice it?"

"I noticed something odd the last couple of showers, but I use a loofah and don't actually touch myself. For some reason today, something told me to check, and there it was. It couldn't have been there too long."

"Poor darling, you must be scared like hell. Have you made an appointment yet?"

"Well, no. I hoped you could come over to be with me when I call. I'm afraid of what they might tell me."

"Give me a half hour. I slept in late. I'll throw on some jeans and a sweater and be right over."

"Monica, you're such as good friend," Devon said. "I don't know what I'd do without you." She started to choke forcing back tears. She ended the call and leaned back to compose herself while she waited.

After the call from Devon, Monica imagined she heard a ripping sound pierce her universe and usher in an overwhelming doom above her head. Her friends considered her the strong one, the reliable one, the empathetic one who absorbed others' emotional pain. That empathetic quality would do her in one of these days, and this episode could be the one to do it. Imogen's breast cancer, then her arrest for killing Henry, Frankie's bizarre mood swings, and now Devon's breast cancer scare, Monica thought how thankful that Fleur was the only other one to have avoided a crisis. Her own crisis, whatever it turned out be, was sure to be on the horizon.

"Now, Imogen, relax like you did this morning and tell me what happened after the dog jumped on you," Davenport said.

"If it's okay with you, I'd like to sit on the chaise."

"Wherever makes you the most comfortable." He shifted his chair so that he was parallel to her.

Session Two

Imogen pressed fingertips on both breasts, and winced from the applied pressure. She knew the soreness came from Roman jumping on her, but she thought the bruising would have gone away after a week, not be worse. Henry was heading toward the bathroom when their eyes met. He did not miss anything when it involved her. She laughed to her friends that his attentiveness after thirty years of marriage was either romantic or frightening.

"What's the matter?" Henry said.

"The bruising hasn't gone away. I think it's worse. Do you think I should see the doctor?"

Henry hesitated before speaking. Imogen found this habit infuriating that he had to process what she said first, unlike her processing as someone spoke to her. Times like this, she wanted to reach down his throat to pull the words out. "Yes."

"A real Liberal with words. That's my Henry."

"You asked me a yes or no question. You didn't ask me to elaborate why, but if that's what you want, I think you might have more than bruising."

"You mean cancer? I had my last mammogram three months ago and it showed nothing unusual."

"Suit yourself. You asked me."

"So you think something's wrong?"

"How should I know? I'm not a doctor, but commonsense says if something unusual begins to happen in your body, get it checked out. It's not like we can't afford medical care."

Imogen looked at him. Henry knew how to manipulate her into doing what he thought she should do, but this time she agreed. "Maybe you're right."

"Of course," he said. Imogen hoped he was wrong, if for no other reason than to tell him so.

Before she opened her eyes, Dr. Davenport said, "Were you and Henry competitive?"

"Not really. I don't find that feminine, or appropriate to compete against my mate. We're strong and weak in different things. I'd say Henry completes me in that he's strong where I'm weak, and vice-versa."

"Well said," Davenport said. "So you didn't argue?"

"Sure we do. I'm not a nitwit without a point of view. That's not the same as competing."

"Of course it isn't. The next session, I'd like to hear about your experience with the diagnosis."

CHAPTER TWELVE

Detective Stokes' ringing telephone jolted him from his concentration. Macy had just stepped out to grab an early lunch for them when he had the call that Fleur Sanders waited downstairs for one of the detectives on the Imogen Vine case. He looked down at his grumbling belly. Food had to wait now. He met her at the elevator and directed her into an interview room.

He remembered the list of Imogen's close friends. Fleur Sanders worked as a buyer for one of the department store chains, divorced, no kids, travelled frequently. By the looks of her and that confident stride, he had no doubt she got what she wanted in life. But she had something more about her that sent a ripple of excitement through him.

"Good morning, Ms. Sanders. We appreciate you coming in to speak to us." Stokes motioned her to have a seat. He seated himself across the table from her.

"I'm glad to do what I can," Fleur said. "We're all distressed over what happened to poor Henry. I just can't make myself believe Imogen would do such a thing."

"You know she's confessed, but we still want to get a picture of their lives together. Any recent disagreements? How did they get along? What about their friends? You know the kind of thing." He did not want to add that they needed a stronger motive in case she recanted her confession. Even with an admission, an attorney like Erin

Fitzgerald could pound holes in their case if they did not have a sound foundation to support their charge.

"I've known Imogen for years. I'd seen her around the non-profit circuit, but we became good friends while we worked on a committee together for some cause or another. I was married at the time, so the four of us had dinner together often. Imogen and Henry had disagreements, but they were more like the nit-picky type of spats most married couples have—like the time Imogen forget to get gas and they ran out on the way to the restaurant to meet us. Henry was steamed, but he'd gotten over it by the end of the evening."

"Can you tell me anything else about their other friends?"

"Well, there's Monica Aames, Devon Bateman, and Frankie Campbell. Monica is probably the closest to Imogen. They go way back. Then there's Dr. Tate—I mean Dr. Tate Marsdon. He became friends after he did reconstruction surgery on Henry after a terrible auto accident." Fleur paused. Stokes thought he saw her eyes grow watery, but she held back. "I feel so bad that he was the one who found Henry. That must've been horrible for him."

"They were that close?"

"Oh, yes. Imogen always said Tate had become more like the sons they never got to see. They have a daughter and two boys, you know."

"Say for the sake of speculation, do you know of anyone Imogen might want to protect?"

That question threw Fleur off balance. Stokes saw confusion and then a startled expression.

"Are you asking me if Imogen would confess to killing Henry to protect someone else?"

"Yes," Stokes said.

Fleur went silent so long that Stokes thought she had decided not to continue.

"I guess she'd do it to protect one of her children. But they're all out of town."

Stokes did not ask the obvious question about the man they considered a son. He wanted her to come up with that conclusion on her own.

"I don't think I understand what you're implying."

"I'm only speculating," Stokes said. "We have an odd situation where the woman confessed to a murder she says she can't remember doing. You've known her a long time. What do you make of that?"

"I can't make anything of that. I find it hard to believe Imogen would kill Henry, but covering up for someone else goes beyond anything I could see happening."

"Like I said, I'm testing the waters. Until she remembers, we need to look at every angle."

"I see. I'll give it some thought." Fleur seemed to notice her surroundings for the first time. "We're in one of those interrogation rooms, aren't we? Are we being taped?"

"Yes, mainly for reference."

"That's too bad," she said. She gave him a sly smile and a wink.

Stokes started to build a fantasy of getting lost in her softness. He shut down his thoughts. He could not do that, at least now. She was a party in an active investigation.

He cleared his throat. "Just one more question, if you don't mind."

"Yes, I'm free tonight."

He knew by the heat on his face that he was blushing. She had charm, he had to admit. He laughed, and said. "Uh, that wasn't my question. How well do you know

Erin Fitzgerald?"

"Not too well. We're on nodding terms because of Tate, but not friends."

"So you wouldn't know anyone with a grudge against her?"

"Heavens no. I guess you're referring to her friend's murder. What a tragic coincidence."

"What coincidence?"

"The she and Tate both lost someone close within days of the other. I didn't know her friend, but I can imagine her grief. And to think she's still able to carry on with her cases."

Stokes thought something was odd about the timing, too.

He escorted Fleur to the elevator, and stood with her until the door opened. Her perfume hovered around her, drawing him back into the fantasy again. When she got into the elevator and faced him, her eyes bore into him over a wide smile. She had a magnetism he did not experience often. *Once this case is over*, was all he could think.

His pulse raced on his way back to his desk. "Where's Macy with that food?"

"I'm here. What's going on?" Macy dumped the bags of lunch on his desk and started to divide their dishes.

"One of Imogen Vine's friends was here—Fleur Sanders."

"Learn anything?"

"Yes, she's a fine-looking woman."

Macy laughed. "That hot, huh?"

"Steaming hot."

"Settle down, boy. Did you learn anything about the case?"

"I suggested Imogen might be covering for someone,

and Fleur thought she'd only do that for one of her kids. But she also said that Henry thought of Dr. Marsdon as a son. It got me to thinking. He's the one that found Henry. He was alone with Imogen all that time before an officer arrived. Plenty of time to prompt Imogen. Remove evidence he overlooked before. Who knows?"

"Something to think about." Macy bit into the large burger.

"I asked her about Erin Fitzgerald. She said she doesn't know her well. We have a common denominator there, too. The doc again."

"Unfortunately, we have more commonalities than him."

"You're right." Stokes raised his sandwich up to his mouth, but the phone rang again, so he answered it. He turned to Macy and said, "Monica Aames and Devon Bateman are here."

"What do we know about them?"

"Monica Aames organizes charity benefits, corporate parties, and destination weekends. Devon Bateman's between jobs, but sells real estate on the side. Both educated, active in the charity circuit. That's how they're connected."

"I'll do their interview. Keep an eye on their reactions. There's got to be one in the group who knows something."

Stokes went into observation with his food, while Macy led the two women into the interview room. Stokes raised his eyebrows at their manner, jittery and apprehensive. They were here to help, not as suspects. He guessed Macy thought the same thing. He sat across from them and waited until they settled into their seats.

"Thanks for coming in," Macy said.

"We want to help Imogen anyway we can," Monica

said. "Except I don't think we understand why you want to see us. As far as we know, Imogen confessed. Isn't that all you need?"

"There's always a concern when someone does not remember the crime they confessed to doing."

Monica gave him a knowing look, "Ah, so you're thinking she has trauma-induced memory loss because she might be a witness to something she thought so awful that she's blocked it out so she doesn't have to deal with it."

Macy smiled, as Stokes did.

"You're very perceptive, Ms. Aames. Until she's positive she knows what happened, we can't close the investigation."

"I see," Monica said. "What can we tell you?"

"Tell me about her life before this happened. Were she and her husband happy?"

"Oh, yes." Monica looked at Devon. "Don't you agree?"

"They argued once in a while, but nothing that lasted long," Devon said.

"The night of the reception, I thought they had one of their tiffs, and Henry stayed home," Monica said. "They were like that, but I never had an idea like they didn't get along."

"What about their family relationships?"

"They have three children, but I'm sure you already know that. All three are married and live in other states." Monica looked at Devon and said, "Right?"

"Oh, yes. They visited each of them a couple of times a year. I think they were a close family, even with the distance."

"What about other close relationships?"

"There's Tate. I mean, Dr. Marsdon," Monica said.

"He and Henry became friends after Henry's accident. The Vines sort of adopted him, you might say. Imogen is very protective over him. She even maneuvered a meeting to introduce him to Erin. She kept saying how a young man like that should have a wife to take care of him. Old-fashioned thinking, of course, but that's the way Imogen is. When she cares for someone, she's never less than a hundred percent."

"I see," Macy said.

Monica did not miss the affirming expression on his face. "What are you thinking? That Imogen is protecting him?"

"I didn't say that."

"But you thought it," Monica said. "First, it's ridiculous to think of any reason Tate would harm Henry. Second, it's beyond belief Imogen would protect anyone who hurt Henry."

"I agree," Devon said. She had straightened up in her chair. "You've got that all wrong. You'd be better off looking at one of us. He put Henry back together after his terrible ordeal. He cared about him. He would never do that."

Macy drew back. Stokes thought that quiet one sure had fire. Maybe he misread her demure presence. He had pegged her as submissive, but she must have another reason, like illness, for her subdued attitude.

"I'm exploring all the possibilities. I'm not accusing anyone," Macy said.

Devon looked appeased, but now had an apprehensive posture. Monica looked amused at Macy's discomfort.

"Anyone else Imogen is close to? I have you," he nodded to Monica. "and Devon. Fleur came in just before you. Anyone else significant?"

"Frankie," Devon said.

"Yes, Frankie Campbell. Actually, Francesca. She and Imogen are closer in age. They've been friends for years, too. She's been going to Imogen with all her problems for most of their friendship."

"Anyone else?"

"None that I can think of, but we're not each other's keepers. Most of us have busy lives. We've only seen so much of one another this week because of Henry's death. Otherwise, it might have been two or more weeks before we had the chance to get together."

"How well do you know Erin Fitzgerald?"

"I know of her," Monica said. "I know she and Tate have been seeing each other several months. She has a great reputation as a defense attorney. She's defending Imogen. I also know that someone killed her best friend a couple days ago. Personally, I barely know her well enough to speak, but that will change since we met her in her office yesterday."

"Oh, I see. Was that case-related?"

"Yes. She asked us if we would come in for a chat about Imogen. She wanted to know more about what's been going on in her life. Not different from the questions you're asking now." Monica turned to Devon. "What about you?"

"I hadn't heard of her until I heard Tate was seeing her. After Monica told me her background, I'm glad she's handling Imogen's case."

"Did Imogen request her, or did Tate ask her to represent her?"

Monica thought a few seconds. "I think she volunteered. We're all grateful for that. I've heard Imogen would've ended up hiring a random attorney who didn't know anything about her. Erin knows her background."

"That's true," Macy said. "Although one could pose

the question about whether she could be impartial."

"An interesting angle, but you don't honestly believe that."

"I'm not ruling out anything."

"Can we go now?" Monica nudged Devon to get up. Stokes observed the distressed expression on Devon's face. She looked drained. Stokes thought she might be sick, after all.

"Sure. We also want to get more background on Imogen's life before this happened. You two have provided that. We appreciate your time."

The two women stood up, and walked out before Macy had a chance to stand up from his chair to escort them. Stokes tapped on the window, and joined Macy in the hallway.

"So what do you think?" Macy said.

"We didn't learn too much more than what we already knew."

"We're getting a definite picture of the doctor's relationship with the Vines. Like a son, Fleur had said. But being that close, what earthly reason could he have to kill his good friend?"

"Let's see what Ms. Campbell has to say. She agreed to come in?"

"Yes, but grudgingly. I can tell she's a real ball-buster."

"Interesting a personality like that fitting in with the women we've met so far. They're assertive, but not aggressive."

"Let's do some checking on the doctor. I have a hunch he figures into this somehow."

Monica watched each friend as she walked into Frankie's restaurant. Frankie had suggested this two o'clock lunch at her restaurant as a respite from the grim events of the past week. The deaths had taken a measure of joy out of them. Their lowered faces expressed the solemnity of a funeral reception more than a light meal with friends.

Monica saw that Devon looked tense—the appointment today probably weighed on her mind. Fleur did not throw herself down in the path of the waiter this time either. Frankie had changed, too—a determination had replaced her usual aggressive attitude. Monica did not understand but attributed her change to unrelated problems at the restaurant.

"I need a drink," Frankie said. She raised her hand up and snapped her fingers. "Ben, get me a drink. Find out what they want while you're at it."

"A terrible week so far," Monica said. "I can't believe any of this is happening." She glanced at Devon who looked on the verge of tears.

"Have you heard anything new about Imogen?" Frankie said.

"I had another call from Erin. She still can't get too much out of her. She starts seeing that psychiatrist. She suggested that one of us might be the friend Imogen is worried about, but that the problem is too embarrassing to mention in front of everyone. She said anything I told her would be confidential. Her only concern is Imogen."

"I got the same call," Frankie said. "What a nerve she has."

"That wasn't meant as an accusation, Frankie," Monica said.

"Well, it's not me," Devon said. "There's no way Imogen could know about…"

"About what," Fleur said.

"I found a lump," Devon said. "It developed fast. To

be honest, I'm petrified. It's different when it's happening to you. I don't want to die, but I don't want to be butchered either."

Monica took her hand and squeezed drawing Devon's eyes to hers. "You won't know anything for certain until we see your doctor. Try not to worry until you're positive you have something to worry about."

"You're right. I'm sorry, everyone. I've had nothing else on my mind since yesterday. Monica, tell them what we can do to help Imogen."

Monica turned to the other women, keeping a tight squeeze on Devon's hand. "Erin believes that if we can sort out what has Imogen so concerned, that she'll relax enough to remember what happened when Henry died. She has no memory of killing Henry but insists she must have. There's always a chance she didn't do it. I think she witnessed the murder, and that traumatized her into a hysterical amnesia."

"That's stretching it, isn't it?" Frankie said.

"Why not? She doesn't remember anything, and that scenario makes a hell of lot more sense than her stabbing Henry to death. They argued, but I never knew either of them to be violent," Monica said. Frankie and her obstructive comments had started to get on her nerves. Monica took a deep breath, sipped her wine, and regrouped. "Listen, all I'm saying is that Erin asked me for help with this girl's identity and her problem that has Imogen so worried. If none of us know anything, then it is what it is."

"What about asking Tate? Maybe she said something before. You know, before he found Henry, I mean," Fleur said.

"She didn't," Frankie said.

"How would you know?" Monica said. "Unless you

were there. Oh, that's it. Frankie was there and saw it all. She's just keeping it all a secret to protect the real murderer."

"You're so funny, we all forgot to laugh," Frankie said.

"Monica," Fleur said, "sarcasm does not become you. That isn't funny at all."

"You're both drunk," Devon said. "Stop bickering. Let's get back to Imogen's problem."

"Maybe it's about Tate," Frankie said. "Imogen told me that Tate was seeing that dead medical student."

"Who?" Fleur demanded.

"The *murdered* medical student. I didn't want to tell Erin for obvious reasons."

"I don't believe it," Fleur said. "He's not the type. Besides, if he knew her, he would admit it."

"Not if he killed her."

Before anyone realized her intention, Monica reached across the table and slapped Frankie so hard across her cheek that she reeled sideways off her chair and then backward onto the floor. Monica pulled out cash from her wallet and threw it on the table. "I'm sorry, but I've had it with this bitch."

Frankie's staff rushed to help her, but Ben was the only one to offer his arm to help her on her feet.

"Get away from me. I can get up on my own." She glared at Fleur and Devon. "You two get out of my restaurant before I have you thrown out."

"Wait for us," Fleur said. She and Devon followed Monica out the front door.

"I'm sorry I caused a scene, guys, but I couldn't take it anymore. She's been a witch the last couple of weeks, but I draw the line when she starts accusing someone of murder. Tate, of all people? Who would believe that?"

"You're right," Fleur said. "I've noticed those

innuendos. Should we tell Tate? It's sounds so childish to say it out loud."

"What could she hope to gain? We're all friends. Maybe she's jealous of us because we're younger," Devon said. Monica and Fleur gave her an endearing look.

"Devon, you have more important concerns than worrying about that old alcoholic."

"Listen," Fleur said. "I'm going to do a little investigating of *Miss Thang* in there. I want to know what alley she's been crawling into. She's up to something nasty. I can feel it in my bones."

"Be careful. I'll call you after Devon sees the doctor."

By the time they arrived for the appointment that afternoon, Devon could not stop shaking. She questioned whether she could ever have Imogen's strength to carry on the treatment.

"Stop thinking the worst," Monica said. "Your problem is that you like to worry in advance of having anything to worry about." They sat alone in the waiting room, their silence magnifying the tension. Devon had not let go of Monica's hand since they sat down twenty minutes ago.

The doctor decided on a needle aspiration to verify his diagnosis of a cyst.

"There are many benign breast conditions, fibrosis and cysts the most common. While the cysts are not cancerous, they can grow or become more sensitive before menstruation. You had your mammogram and an MRI last month. I see the reason for the MRI was this tiny area," he pointed to the film on the light box. "The procedure I'm going to do is called aspiration. It's not too uncomfortable and doesn't take long either. The nurse will help prepare you."

"Can my friend stay?"

"Absolutely. And don't worry. This could be a case of a fluid-filled cyst that needs to be drained. If that's the case, once the fluid is gone, the cyst will collapse, and the lump disappear."

"God, I hope so," Devon said. It took all her energy to suppress the flow of tears.

Once the doctor stood in place next to her, Devon relaxed. She held on to Monica's hand on the opposite side of the table and kept her eyes locked on Monica's soft expression. The hands of the doctor grasped her breast, searching for and isolating the area with the lump. Devon worried she might throw up, but when she felt the needle go through the skin and penetrate an area deep inside, she let out a sigh. She had more discomfort than pain. Not so bad after all.

She moved her head slowly toward the doctor's face. He squinted his eyes, concentrating on his task. She had no words to describe the relief when he began to use the syringe.

"Yes, young lady. You have a cyst. After we get rid of the fluid, you'll be fine. No other treatment should be necessary unless the cyst fills again. If that happens, come back in and we'll do this again.

Devon started crying in convulsive sobs. She never thought a big cyst could be a good thing.

"Try to calm yourself. I'm not done yet."

"I'm sorry," Devon said. "Those were such beautiful words." She looked over at Monica, who had watery eyes of her own. She smiled down at Devon and patted her hand.

Devon walked with shaky knees on the way to Monica's car. Her erratic emotions left her lightheaded.

"I still say that you scared the doctor when you wouldn't let go of him," Monica said.

"I don't care. I'm so relieved after being scared out of my mind with fear, that I could've hugged the pieces out of everyone in the office.

"Finally, something good coming out of a crisis," Monica said. "Think of how happy Imogen will be to hear your news. I hope her crisis ends this well."

"Good morning, Doctor," Imogen said.

"Good morning, Imogen," Davenport said. "Did you have a good night?"

"Yes, I did. I think I'm feeling stronger. My thoughts are sharper."

"Good. You left off telling me about Henry suggesting you see a doctor for the soreness in your breasts. Would you like to talk more about that?"

"I would, actually. From the beginning to the final reconstruction, I don't believe I had any thoughts except for the right now. I didn't go back and think, wow, did that just happen? Or how did I get through it? Telling you about it puts the ordeal into time perspective. It took up all my thoughts, my past and present until I couldn't think of anything else ever happening around me. Does that make sense?"

Session Three

"I'll try to put this in simple terms. We're doing a breast MRI today. That stands for magnetic resonance imaging. What that means is we'll take a computerized picture linked to a magnet. We'll be able to look at your problem areas from every angle in virtually hundreds of images. I'll read the results and pass it on to Dr. Clarendon. Do you have any questions for me before we get started?"

"Is there radiation?"

"No. This is a benefit of this procedure. A breast MRI is new technology that has proven to detect cancer that might not be visible on a mammogram. We don't use them in a routine breast exam, but that might change. Some patients are opposed to radiation exposure. Any other concerns?"

"I guess not," Imogen said. "Except that you really need to do something about your decorating style." Granted medical facilities are required to be sterile, but someone needed to address these greyish white walls. How awful for that color to be the last thing you saw before you died. She felt on the verge of a crying spell, but tightened her facial muscles and closed her eyes. Not now. Later.

"Relax, Mrs. Vine. No one has ever suffered on my table," the technician said.

Imogen positioned herself face down on the scanning table. When her breasts were secure in the hollow in the table, which encased coils to detect the magnetic signal, she held back the impulse to escape. Before she had time to process her call to action, the table moved into a tunnel-like machine. She held her breath until she thought she would faint.

After the initial series of images, the technician gave Imogen a contrast agent intravenously, and assured her that it was not radioactive. "We use this sometimes to improve the visibility if there is a tumor." The technician took several more images.

"We're all done. That wasn't so bad, was it?"

The process took no more than thirty minutes, but

seemed like ten hours. All she wanted to do now was to get home to Henry and a hot bath, together or separately.

Erin waited in her office for the detectives. She jumped when Penny spoke through the intercom that they had arrived.

"Send them in, please."

She had participated in these interviews before, but not as a victim. They would be the ones asking the questions, discerning facts in the offhand way of conversation. She would be leveling each statement for content to be sure she said the right things, answered succinctly, gaged her answers on a scale of importance. Yes, she had an anxious flutter of nerves.

Penny opened the door and motioned for the two detectives to enter Erin's office. She could have met with them in the conference room, but she wanted absolute focus for the personal nature of this interview. The men sat in the two chairs facing her desk.

"Can I get either of you anything, water, coffee, tea?" Penny waited until she saw them shake their heads, and closed the door behind her.

"Have you had any progress, Detectives?"

"Unfortunately, no. We've had news from the toxicology report that they determined the poison used was hemlock," Macy said.

"Hemlock? Like the poison Socrates drank?"

"The same," Macy said. "It appears to have been in the water bottles. The remaining three bottles were loaded with the stuff."

"What water? I hadn't had time to shop. Actually, I drank my last one on the way to work."

"You're certain?" Stokes said.

"Yes. I might not be Suzy Homemaker, but I know what I have on hand."

"If you're positive about that," Stokes said, "we have to assume that someone dropped them off after you left for work. We learned from neighbors that Hermione took off for a run and didn't return for over an hour. They didn't see anyone go to your place, but one neighbor thought she saw something on your door. Our perp could have sneaked up, left without being observed. We can check for traffic cams and neighborhood security surveillance, but you get a lot of traffic. Without knowing what we're looking for, the search could be tedious."

"So, you believe someone wanted me dead, and Hermione took the bullet for me?"

"That's a way of looking at it," Macy said. "Did you have any luck thinking of anyone who holds a grudge against you, a disgruntled client, or maybe an employee of your firm?"

"No, detective. There isn't anyone so far."

"We have some other questions that might seem irrelevant or intrusive, but we need the information for the Henry Vine case. This could border on a conflict of interest for you," Macy said.

A sense of defiance sprung up in Erin, a reaction she had monitored and advised clients on many times. "Go on."

"You've known Tate Marsdon for several months, we understand," Macy said.

"Yes, that's correct."

"You've observed his relationship with the Vines. Would you say the Vines thought a great deal of him, and he felt the same way about them?"

"Yes. Your point?"

"We've heard from Imogen's friends that Henry and

Imogen thought of him as a son."

"Yes. I still don't see where you're going with these questions."

"Maybe Imogen is lying. Maybe she knows the murderer, but her loyalty prevents her from exposing the person."

"Balderdash," Erin said. That's your new working theory? Where's your motive?"

Macy took a breath. "We don't know yet. But we have to look at anyone who spent time with the couple the days leading up to murder."

"If this is the best you can come up with, I'd rather take my chances in court defending Imogen. I guess you want to pin Hermione's murder on him too, even though he has multiple witnesses to confirm his alibi during that time she was murdered. I think we're done here."

Macy and Stokes looked at each other before rising to leave. Stokes said, "We'll keep you posted about any developments in both cases."

Erin almost choked on her rage like a switch went off inside her head. She turned her back on them. *Let them find their own way out.* She had to get air before the world crashed down on her head and suffocated her. She grabbed her purse, keys, and phone, and ran down the hallway to the stairs past Penny's desk.

"I need a break. I'll be back later."

She left Penny with mouth dropped open and shock expression. Whatever she wants to tell me can wait.

Session Four

Imogen sat on the examination table, stripped down to her panties, except for the paper gown, sterile, crisp and white, draped around her shoulders, open at the front.

Not until the doctor walked through the door, did she realize her anxiety. She wrapped her arms across her breasts and waited for her to speak.

"Mrs. Vine. I'm Dr. Clarendon, your oncologist. I'm happy to meet you," she said, extending her hand. "I can understand you're apprehensive, but be assured we will make this process as comfortable as possible. I reviewed the results of your mammograms and ultrasound ordered by your GP, and the breast MRI that I ordered for you."

Imogen knew her pause was an attempt to measure her words and soften the bad news. "Go ahead, please. I just want to hear the words, good or bad."

"First, what you have is termed DCIS, a pre-invasive breast cancer confined to the milk ducts. DCIS stands for 'ductal carcinoma in situ,' where abnormal cells are found in the lining of breast ducts. To give you a perspective, its classification is Stage 0, less risky than the Stages I-IV, Stage IV being the worst. Your lymph nodes status is negative, free of breast cancer cells. The pathologist sent his report. He classified your tumors as Grade 1, meaning the breast cancer cells are closer to normal cells and have a slow growth rate. I sent a tissue sample from the biopsy we performed last week, for a genomic testing called Oncotype DX DCIS Score, or DCIS Score. The test looks at groups of genes and how active they are within the tumor. This testing provides the likelihood of recurrence of breast cancer within ten years based on a scale of 0-100. Your score was 49."

"So that means, what, a fifty-fifty chance?"

"We have developed a hormonal treatment plan after surgery. A drug called Tamoxifen for breast cancers that are estrogen receptor-positive. You've said you're opposed to radiation and chemotherapy, so this is one part of your personal treatment plan. The other part involves an appropriate diet and low consumption of alcohol. I can't say we won't suggest chemo later, but we can start with this strategy."

"So the tumors have to be removed. I've heard that some women are having double mastectomies to avoid cancer in the other breast, or having the surgery before they're diagnosed based on family history. I want to talk to my husband first, but I've settled my mind to do both. This experience has frightened the wits out of me. I don't want to take the chance of going through this a second time."

"That's understandable. That's a decision I made for myself when my sister and mother were diagnosed."

Imogen had to take a long look at the other woman's chest, fascinated that she had a more than ample bust size.

"I recommend reconstruction for you, too. It's important for a woman to feel womanly and desirable. None of this will be a walk in park, but you have a good support system. That's important to keep up your morale. For the reconstruction, I have names of plastic surgeons for referral."

"My husband is good friends with Dr. Marsdon, so I'll go to him."

"He's one of the doctors on this list. You'll be in good hands."

CHAPTER THIRTEEN

Tate thought of himself as a man of action. This hesitation, his avoidance had to be a product of the emotional trauma of the last few days. He decided to approach this as any other personal challenge. It was true that anyone experiencing distress should avoid major decisions. On the other hand, business was business.

He brought in a bottle of water and twisted off its cap. He sipped more than drank as he contemplated the exchange he planned with Derren. In a sudden burst of determination, he drank the rest of the water, tossed the empty aside, and reached for his cell phone to send Derren a text for an urgent meeting.

He pulled out the copied receipts from the other day. He had found more charges buried under other accounts on the income statement. His eyes rolled over the figures again. Neither of them had gone to a convention, seminar, or class that required travel, yet he saw over five thousand dollars in travel and about as much in meals. He tried to take a clinical approach to his own distress, but he lost the battle.

Tate looked at his surgeon's hands, shaking. He subdued his temper as he had learned to do from childhood. He was dangerous that way. Holding back rage only worked well for so long before it exploded, like steam under pressure. Life had been fair to him so far, and his exposure to con men had been nonexistent. He had a hard choice choosing what bothered him more, being robbed or being somebody's fool.

Rachelle had gone home at three, so when the door opened and he heard footsteps, he knew Derren had arrived. He swaggered up to Tate's office door and leaned in.

"Hey, Bud. What's up?"

Tate frowned. "Don't call me Bud. Come in and have seat. I need to speak with you."

"Chill out, man. You're much too uptight. Everything's serious with you."

"Like embezzlement?"

Derren's face went pale, but he recovered at once. "What d'you mean?

"I mean like these travel and meals expenses. Like this advertising expense. Seven thousand dollars? I want an explanation."

"Listen, man. You're getting this all wrong. This is for the both of us."

"Our partnership agreement states that no expenses, over occupancy costs and medical supplies, are allowed unless we both sign off on them. Exactly what kind of advertising is this? And where're all the new patients?"

"You're so wrong, man. You're going to feel bad when you know what a sweet deal I got us."

Tate did not break eye contact. Derren cowered under the stare but held his stance.

"Listen, I bought air time for two-minute segments on one of the television stations. It's in production now." Derren flushed, his forehead at the moist beginning of beads of sweat.

"That doesn't explain the secrecy. That doesn't explain

why I haven't seen a contract. Or why you paid in cash."

"That was part of the deal, man. Discount for cash. I think the station owner is going through a divorce."

"I want to see a contract to support what you're saying. And there'll be no commercial airing on any station until I see it first. Now what about the meals and travel?"

"Just the everyday sort of thing. Taking patients and their friends out for dinner to drum up business. For instance, I provided a paid vacation for a couple who both had cosmetic surgery. They referred two other couples for similar procedures."

"Are you sure the *friends* of these gifts aren't doctors as payment for referring their patients to you?"

"That would only be a coincidence," Derren said.

"Kickbacks, huh. May I remind you that the phrase 'knowing and willful conduct' is broadly interpreted, and you can't claim ignorance of the law as a defense?"

"I think you're overreacting. What benefits me benefits you, too. I get the kids—you get the parents."

"I need to speak with my attorney to find out my exact exposure and compliance issues."

Derren narrowed his eyes into a laser-like glare but said nothing.

The pounding in Tate's chest beat so loudly that he had difficulty hearing his own voice. "Disguising your personal expenses as business deductions means you're stealing from me. I want all the money back in the general account."

Derren turned from barely apologetic to angry and aggressive. "I'm not paying back shit. This is just as much mine is it is yours, and if I want to take out money, I will."

"Then the accountants will apply those expenditures

to your drawing account."

"Try it. I don't have to take being treated like a ten-year old. I didn't do anything wrong, and I won't stand for you making accusations against my integrity."

"Suit yourself. You have until Friday to clear this up. And don't forget the advertising contract and its invoice." Tate held his own version of a caustic stare on Derren until he turned and walked out.

Tate relaxed when he heard him slam the front office door on his way out. Tate considered their partnership was broken. He flipped through the contacts on his phone for his attorney. No answer, but he left a call back message. He leaned back in his chair, his body at rest for the first time since Derren entered the office. "At least," he muttered, "that's one confrontation behind me."

Fleur had been so angry with Frankie that she thought she might be capable of killing the woman. Frankie's accusations had a dismissive quality, finality to their relationship, albeit tenuous, the five of them had shared the last several years. Fleur suspected someone else behind Frankie's rant. A boyfriend? Granted, they tended to view Frankie's ambition and zeal for work her constant lover, but even a woman of steel has needs. Nothing wrong with that, right? But what if Frankie involved herself with someone nasty or plain dangerous? Fleur admitted that she had no other inkling to explain Frankie's behavior, but she had a plan to find out.

With a thermos of coffee and a bag of cheese puffs, Fleur sat across from Frankie's restaurant concealed behind other cars in the parking lot. After their meeting this afternoon, she had borrowed her neighbor's nephew's black Miata. Now, with her hair pulled up under a sweater cap, she sat calmly waiting to follow Frankie once she closed for the night. She never allowed anyone else to close the place, worried about employee theft, so no guesswork at where Frankie would be right now. If she kept a couple of blocks back, she would have no problem finding out what Frankie got up to at night. An adrenalin jolt ripped through her midsection when Frankie closed the heavy metal door and slid into her black Lexus.

Frankie pulled out onto the street. Fleur drank in the intoxicating cocktail of anticipation, danger, and determination when Frankie's car stopped at the red traffic light two blocks away. Fleur turned on her engine, flipped on her lights, and shifted into first gear. She waited. When she saw the light turn green, she maneuvered her car in Frankie's direction.

The darkness of the Phoenix neighborhoods beyond the major arteries gave the streetlights a bright contrast. Fleur started to worry her car would stand out in the sparse traffic, but set that idea aside when Frankie turned east instead of heading north to her house. This was it. She was going to find out on her first try. Maybe she should consider becoming a private detective. This was easy.

Frankie pulled into a driveway. Fleur kept her pace within the speed limit, and passed by the house. She drove down to a roundabout, turned around and looked for a parking spot. Casual cars did not park in this neighborhood, so she pulled under a low-hanging mesquite that concealed her car in the darkness. She slid out into the cold winter air and pressed the car door closed until the inside light went out. This had to be quick. Parking here did not guarantee that a neighbor passing by would not spot her car and report it to the police. These residents knew their environment, so the odds were that someone would notice before she got back. She had to take the chance. Her tightly wound nerves made her brave and probably reckless.

The occupants of the homes in this area prided themselves on sustaining the desert environment. That meant no sidewalks, grass, decorative water features, and best of all, no overhead street lighting, Fleur backtracked in the cool darkness until she found Frankie's parked car. Once she had a good look at the house, she recognized it as a place she had visited before.

I don't believe it. I have to get a peek inside to make sure I'm right.

Fleur reckoned the darkness gave her the courage. Her plan had been to find out if Frankie had a mystery man, but she had not expected the exhilaration of discovery on her first outing. After what happened today, Fleur had to have proof or no one would believe her. She winced as her sneakers crunched on impact with the crushed granite driveway. She stopped to listen. No sounds from inside or outside. She got closer. She pulled out her phone to make sure she turned it on silent and pushed the button to activate the camera. One photo, that's all she needed. Then, she would show Monica and that hunky cop.

She reached the top of the driveway, moving toward the glow from one of the windows. She tiptoed, her eyes fixed on the light. She heard a sound behind her, and jerked her head around. She caught a brief glimpse of Frankie's face before she felt the impact of the cricket bat strike her face.

Detective Macy got the call to a possible murder scene at three in the morning. A battered woman left for dead in a parking lot at a medical facility on McDowell Road. She had looked dead enough at first glance when they called it in, but the officer who found her noticed a weak pulse and called for an ambulance.

"What did the paramedics say?" Macy asked the officer.

"He couldn't say. From her injuries, I'd say someone hit her multiple times in the face, the back, and legs. Pretty gruesome. She must be a fighter to still be breathing. They're expecting to talk with you."

"What made them call *me*?"

"Joe thought she looked familiar from one of your current cases and thought there might be a connection. He worked on the initial interviews for the Henry Vine murder, but he couldn't remember her name. She needed immediate medical attention, so he told the paramedics to take her in as a Jane Doe until someone established her identity."

Macy went silent to think through this development. If the wife confessed, and they weren't looking at other suspects, maybe this had nothing to do with that crime. Still, was there such a thing as a second and third coincidence? After the ass chewing he and Stokes received from Erin this afternoon, he decided to take a gentler approach. He would not let go of Marsdon's possible involvement, but he had to keep an open mind for other possibilities. First, he needed this woman's identity.

Monica jumped at the sound of her cell phone. Probably a wrong number. *Better check who's calling anyway.* She looked down at the small screen for the time, and when she saw Tate's private number, she pushed the green button. "Yeah! Sorry, I mean, hello."

"Monica, I need you to come to the hospital right away. It's Fleur. Someone attacked her. She had no identification on her so the paramedics brought her in as a Jane Doe a few minutes ago. I'm here for another trauma case, so they pulled me over for an evaluation, and I recognized her. She's in bad shape, but the trauma doctor said she'll make it. I know she doesn't have any family in town, and she has you listed as her emergency contact at my office. She's going to need your support when she comes around."

"My God. How horrible. I'll be there as soon as I can. Will you still be there?" A wave of helplessness, loss of control, fear, panic, rushed over her and pushed her backward into her pillow. She did not know if she was strong enough to do this alone.

"I'm due in surgery on the other patient in five minutes. I'll check with you while Fleur's getting ready for me."

"Thank God."

She thought he must be able to read minds when he said, "All you need to do is be here for her when she comes around. We'll do the rest. Try to stay calm."

"Ok, see you later," Monica said. She had to hold back the tears until she got him off the line.

Monica dropped the phone on the bed and rushed to dress in yesterday's clothes. She pulled her hair under a ball cap, grabbed her purse and keys, and ran out. She arrived at the emergency room entrance disoriented and nauseated. What was happening? Her world had started collapsing around her with no reason. Before she found the right person to ask about Fleur, she turned around to find Detective Macy watching her.

"What are you doing here?" Monica said. On top of

her distress over Fleur, his presence irritated her.

"She's in good hands right now. Still in surgery for her internal injuries," he said. "Let's move over to a quiet corner and talk."

Once they sat, he said, "The officers on the scene recognized her from Imogen's case and called me. We never know when an incident is related. The attack might have nothing to do with Imogen, but we don't like to overlook obvious coincidences."

Monica's back straightened. Her emotional fog lifted, and her mental acuity returned. "You think there might be a connection? If you think this has something to do with Imogen, I need to tell you what happened today, I mean, yesterday now."

Macy saw her eyes following an internal video. "I had a nasty scene with Frankie. We met for lunch. All of us were upset about Imogen and then Devon's health issue, when out of nowhere Frankie started rattling off some crap about Tate having a secret affair with the murdered med student." Monica took a deep breath. "You'll find out anyway, so I'll admit I slapped Frankie across the face. I hope I broke her nose. With all our circle has been through recently, none of us wanted to hear crazy talk. Fleur told Devon and me that she was determined to find out what Frankie was playing at. When we left the restaurant, I went to the doctor with Devon, and Fleur drove off fired up."

"Is Fleur the type to play private detective? In other words, would she, say, follow Frankie?"

"That never occurred to me before, but yes she would. That's one way of figuring out Frankie's game."

"Fleur traded vehicles with someone yesterday evening. Officers found that car up on Durango Cliffs Drive in response to a complaint call from a property owner. You know the neighborhood? Someone who didn't know about the switch would have no reason to connect Fleur with this car. He or she dumped her miles away believing there'd be no connection to this area."

Monica shut her eyes tight. "Wait a minute," she said. "Tate's partner lives up there. Derren Davide. I remember the house from when he hosted a Christmas party for all their patients last year."

"What about Tate? He lives around there?"

"I haven't been to his place, but I know he lives in the towers off Scottsdale Road."

Macy tapped his pencil on his notepad, eyes fixed in a meditative trance. He startled Monica when he said, "Right. I'm getting the picture. Monica, thank you for sharing this information. I believe we can piece together what happened to Fleur."

"What can I do? Maybe I could ask some of her staff. Find out if they know anything strange going on."

He gave her a sharp look. He opened his mouth to speak, looked like he thought better of it, and then chose his words in a fatherly tone. "Be patient. Don't try to be a hero. What happened to your friend is what happens when amateurs insert themselves into a police investigation. And don't go out alone. When you leave here, get a security guard to walk you to your car. We're guessing about what might be happening, but we could be wrong. Someone else could have attacked Fleur for an unrelated reason. Until we know, don't take any chances."

Monica shook his hand and watched him walk to the nurses' station, exchange words with the nurse, and leave. As bossy as he was, she surprised herself by wishing he had stayed. A part of her wanted to run out and beg him not to leave her alone. But not her. Too much a sign of weakness.

She needed to get a grip. She leaned back in her chair and rested her feet on a stack of newspapers on a side table she had pulled in front of her. She tapped the screen on her phone to find her book reader app and began to read to pass the time.

Monica had fallen asleep on one of the cushioned chairs. Few people lingered long in the waiting room this time of the night. The walk-ins, processed and led into curtained cubicles, spoke in muted, indistinguishable tones. Hospital personnel, identifiable more from their actions than by uniforms. Monica woke to see the blur of blue scrubs passing in her peripheral vision and sat up. In spite of her thick cardigan and heavy riding boots, she shivered from a cold draft. Where was Tate? A panic rushed over her that she had missed something important while she slept. She looked to the nurses' desk for a friendly face and rested her eyes on an older woman who smiled back at her.

"Any news on my friend yet?"

"Nothing yet, but that's not bad news," Nurse Anne Morrow said.

"What about Dr. Marsdon? Is he still in surgery, too?"

"I'm afraid so. Why not visit the cafeteria and eat something? At least have a cup of coffee. That'll restore you and make the time pass quicker. I'll page you if there's news while you're gone."

"You're right. I need the distraction," Monica said. "Thank you."

Anne Morrow pointed the way to the cafeteria, sending Monica through a series of hallways to the elevator and then down one floor. The monotony of walking through an institutional environment always put her in a hypnotic state, moving forward with unseeing eyes, and no awareness of surroundings. Maybe the reason for that had to do with the circumstances more than environment. Only employees of a hospital came here for reasons other than illness, trauma, or disease— the depressing nature of the clinical culture.

Walking energized her. Like now, the rhythmic movements and the stimulated leg muscles awakened her senses, brightened her disposition, and increased her cognitive skills. Enjoying her return to centeredness, she responded with a springier step when she turned the next corner, and saw the cafeteria door in view. Half way down the hall, she caught movement out of the corner of her eye and turned to look. She saw Dr. Davide bandaging his own right forearm, his skinned knuckles exposed for a short time before he wrapped gauze over the injuries.

Monica wanted to scream, and fought back the impulse to run for her life. Her stomach lurched. She kept moving, praying he had not seen her looking at him. Within steps of the cafeteria, two nurses opened the door from the inside and walked through. She stepped aside to let them pass, giving her the opportunity to look back. She did not see him. She hoped that he had been too occupied with his bandaging task to notice her. She reached for her cell phone, but saw it had no service.

She looked inside the cafeteria, looked down at her phone. The rumbling hunger pangs answered the question of what to do first. As long as she stayed around people in a public area like this, he would not dare harm her. She would call Macy after she ate.

CHAPTER FOURTEEN

Imogen leaned up on her elbows from the prone position she liked during her sessions. Not apprehensive as she had been when they first began, she left with a warm glow of pleasant memories each time. Remembering her life in swatches, though frustrating, had taught her to appreciate what she had more than she did as she lived through each episode. She thought of Henry. How they could fight, and wow, when they loved each other. The arguments stayed vague, but the tender moments flooded over her until she wanted to grab the air to pull them back to her and make them happen again. She would never have a relationship like that with anyone else.

"Dr. Davenport, I believe going back and reliving these memories makes me stronger every day."

"With memories so much of what defines all of us, I would guess recollecting your past year to be empowering. You've gotten through the worst part of your cancer surgery. Tell me about the reconstruction."

Imogen smiled and leaned back, more relaxed than she had been since her treatment started.

Session Five

Imogen wanted to open her eyes. She scrunched her face, struggling to look through her long eyelashes. A blurry individual hovered over her asking if she were awake. By the time she opened her eyes, she recognized Dr. Tate.

"Am I alright?"

"I hope so," he said. "I just operated on you."

"If you're joking around, I must be fine. Is Henry here?"

"He's been here the whole time. I've already spoken to him about how to take care of you. I might check up on how he's doing, if I get an offer for some of your special barbecue."

"Check up on *him*?"

"Of course. You'll be treated like a princess. He'll be taking care of your every need for the next two weeks. You'll exhaust him."

"You men stick together, don't you?" Imogen laughed in spite of the intensity of chest pain. She wanted to ask if this was the worst of the pain, but thought she might not want to know.

"After the nurse checks out a few things, Henry will be right in. I have another surgery, so I have to go. I'll be around to check on you later this afternoon."

Imogen reached over to squeeze his hand, overcome with a sudden surge of emotion. "Thank you."

"My privilege," he said, winking.

"I don't know how I would've gotten through this without you. And Henry, of course, but mainly you, Doc"

She watched him leave, stifling what she knew had to be drug-induced melancholy. She had every reason to thank God that he and Henry had become friends after Henry's accident. Perhaps the heavy medication exaggerated her emotions, the gratitude, good fortune, and comparative relief. All she had to do was lean back and will her body to heal for the next two weeks.

When she returned to her room, Imogen learned her attorney was here to see her. "Who is that, again?" she asked the nurse.

"Miss Erin Fitzgerald."

"Oh, yes. I remember. I know her."

The nurse took her elbow and guided her to a bright room at the end of the corridor opposite the nurse's station.

Imogen backed up when Erin tried to hug her, but regretted it as soon as she did it. "I'm sorry, Erin. I haven't been myself."

"I know you've been through a lot, but you're looking better today."

"Dr. Davenport has been helping me. I know enough to remember you now. How is Tate?"

"As well as can be expected. I mean, worrying about you."

"What a sweet boy," Imogen said, her voice trailing off as the last time she saw Erin.

"Imogen, I want to know if you recall which of your friends needs help. You were quite concerned about her the last time I saw you."

Imogen stared off for a minute, frustrated. "I don't know yet. Dr. Davenport said my memory is returning quickly. I expect the rest will come soon. I know whatever the problem, it was urgent."

"As long as you're getting better, that's the important thing. We need your mind clear so we can concentrate on your defense."

"Erin, do you think Tate would come to see me?" Imogen saw Erin's hesitation and winced. "He hates me, doesn't he?"

"I can't speak for him, but I can ask him to visit. We need to get permission for visitors, so we'll see about that.

I'll see if Dr. Davenport is available when I leave."

"I'm worried about him. I'm uneasy about something. It'll come to me, I guess, but if I could see him, I might remember."

"Okay, Imogen. Is there anything else you need?"

"No,"

"I'll be back tomorrow afternoon. Call my office if you think of anything and can't reach me on my cell."

Imogen sighed and walked to the window to stare, suddenly overwhelmed by fatigue. The confusion she experienced still frightened her. For the first time in her life, she knew what loneliness meant—total isolation inside a closed shell that no one could penetrate. Without Henry, she wanted to die. That possibility was not an option. She had hurt her children too much already. Those people who take their own lives are cowards, and she would not leave that legacy. She would make herself strong, and if she got to that point of wanting to escape life, she would show her children how to be strong and accept responsibility for her actions.

She looked down at the traffic moving at the pace of toy trains, and then on the parking lot south of the facility. She stared at the white coats walking to and from their cars. Not much more than watching pinball while someone else plays, she smiled, but a passive interest to occupy her thoughts. A heavy woman rolled a child in a leg cast in a wheelchair to her car. A man reached inside his back seat and came out carrying a large bouquet of flowers. A couple walked in rhythm but far apart. Two men in suits shook hands before going to different cars. A small girl ran out into the parking lot, her mother flapping her arms to signal her to stop.

Imogen thought how reassuring the passing of time, the flow of life. She wanted to be back with the rest of world to experience it all again through new eyes. She breathed in and let out a loud sigh. She blinked to moisten her eyes before turning back to watch. This time, she saw a tall blond man in a white coat, walking briskly from around the side of the building instead of from the front entrance. His pace caught her attention over the others milling about around the cars, so she kept her eyes on him. When he reached his vehicle, a sporty coupe that looked like dark grey, he unlocked his door but did not get in.

Imogen wished she had her opera glasses or binoculars. Something rang familiar about him. As if for Imogen's amusement, he stood next to his car and looked in every direction. He's agitated, she thought, but why. Then she realized he was talking to someone already inside the car. She saw him pointing to the building and then inside the car. The more she squinted, the more details came into view. He had bandages on one of his hands. He pointed to it with the other hand. He stabbed the air with his finger aimed at the person inside the car.

This is getting good, Imogen smiled. Better than reality television.

In an unexpected move, he stretched out his arm to his side, pointing his forefinger at the street. His head stayed fixed to the inside of the car. He stopped moving, but kept his arm extended. Then he relaxed his body, grabbed the door handle, and released a panel that swung open. Then Imogen saw the same door movement on the passenger side. Oh, great. I get to see the target of his wrath.

First, all she could make out of the woman was her full dark blonde or light brown hair. The woman stood and turned back around to face him, but he ignored her and slid into the driver's seat. Imogen could not make out what happened next, but the woman looked like she tried to catch something and missed. The passenger door closed, and then he drove off, leaving her there. The woman knelt to the ground retrieving small objects. *Oh, I get it. He tossed her purse. What a jerk!*

Imogen recognized her own personality for the first time since *it* happened, but that familiarity brought something else. She watched the woman, bent over, defeated, humiliated, retrieving her belongings with no more dignity than a homeless person scrambling for pennies on the sidewalk. Imogen felt her pain. Wanted to console her. The woman had something familiar about her that appealed to Imogen's empathetic nature.

The woman stood up, looked around, Imogen guessed apprehensive that someone might recognize her, and then pulled her handbag strap over her shoulder. Her hair blew around her head, and she raised her hand to tame the hair and looked upward while she performed the impromptu grooming.

Imogen gasped. *No, this can't be. I know her. What's her name? Shoot. Why can't I remember? Wasn't this her friend?*

Imogen could not explain her anxiety. Seeing this woman frightened her, but felt familiar at the same time. That didn't make sense, she thought. She backed away from the window. She no longer felt the anonymity of an observer. More like a spy caught red-handed in the enemy camp. She wanted to go back to her room where she knew she could lock the door. She hurried down the hallway and stopped at the nurse's station.

"Mrs. Vine, what can I do for you?"

"Please call Dr. Davenport right away. I need to see him. Tell him I remembered something important. Please. It's urgent."

CHAPTER FIFTEEN

Detective Macy and his partner, Martin Stokes, were viewing the surveillance tapes provided by the parking garage company that serviced the airport. Thousands of people passed through this area every day, but just their luck, or the killer's intention, they found no footage near the murdered girl's parked vehicle.

"They sent everything, I hope," Macy said to the technician running the tapes for them.

"Yes, sir."

"Let's take a look at the entrances into the garage, not just where the shuttle drops off their passengers. Set it up on a continuous play so I can replay and rewind on my own. You know me with electronics."

"Yes, sir." Macy saw Stokes give the technician a sidelong glance and a friendly snicker.

"So how do you have it figured so far," Stokes said. He leaned in to watch the screen with an eye on the time stamp.

"The care this guy took to conceal himself makes me think premeditated, but that could be a fortunate coincidence for a crime of passion. From what I've learned, she was a bright girl, beautiful, charismatic, but more book smart than street smart. Not a lot of experience with men, so probably gullible for a slick operator."

Martin paused the tape and leaned back in his chair.

Macy stared at the frozen screen. He knew Martin was preparing the "lecture" he gave when he believed his partner took a murder personally.

"I'm fine. But too many senseless deaths so close together and not one solved."

"Hey, you're not the only detective here. Some of us do manage to solve cases without you."

"Let's find this bastard. He's been caught on film. It's spotting him that's the work."

Before Stokes hit the play button, another officer walked up. "Excuse me, but there's a woman downstairs who says she has information on the Jenny Marcus case. I put her in Interrogation Room One. Video on."

Stokes exchanged looks with Macy. "Hmm, things are looking up."

Macy looked at the woman sitting on the metal chair leaning on her elbows, chin cupped in both palms, staring at the white wall in front of her. Did he know her? He had seen her recently, but where?

"Detective Steve Macy. My partner, Martin Stokes. We're detectives working this case. Do we understand you have information concerning the death of Jenny Marcus?"

"Yes. My name is Francesca Campbell. I normally don't like to get involved, but I felt I should tell what I know. I've been in shock since I heard about it on the news."

Martin took the lead, "What's your information?"

"Well," she said. "Dr. Tate Marsdon was having a relationship with Jenny Marcus. He was her mentor through the school."

"How did you come by this information?" Martin said.

"He told me."

"Just like that?"

"No, not *just* like that. You see, he confided all this to Henry Vine. Henry told Imogen and she told me. He told her before her murder. I'm not *saying* he killed her, but I thought you wanted information on her mystery man."

Macy remembered where he heard that name. "Does he know you're here? I mean, won't this create a bit of a trust issue between the two of you? I thought all of you were friends, Monica, Imogen, Fleur, and your Dr. Tate."

Frankie shifted back in her seat, crossing her arms, and looked up into Stokes' eyes. "Excuse me for trying to do the right thing."

Macy took over in his avuncular manner, "We appreciate when the public comes forward. We solve many cases that way. My partner is curious, as I am, why you would betray your friend to implicate him in a murder case. Many individuals clog up the justice system with false accusations to get even with someone."

"I'm afraid. If he killed her, why wouldn't he kill me? This gives me protection."

Macy and Stokes both stood. Frankie hesitated before rising. "Is that it?"

"Unless you have more information, we'll take it from here. We appreciate you coming in, Ms. Campbell. The officer will escort you back downstairs."

Macy and Stokes followed her out, and then returned to their desks.

"We have to follow up but I'm not buying it," Stokes said. "Did you notice the scratches on her forearms? She doesn't seem to be the type to spend her time gardening."

"Damn it," Macy said. "It just came to me where I've seen her. She tried to get into see Imogen when we first took her into custody."

"Curious too that Erin Fitzgerald is defending Imogen, and is the current 'public' love interest of our new suspect, Dr. Marsdon. More curious that Ms. Fitzgerald's best friend is one of our other murder victims, Hermione Jones. Maybe the doctor killed both of them to cover up his murder. But we need to look at Ms. Campbell. She also has a connection to all three cases. I'll check out the doc's background, his practice, his financials, and the works. I have a feeling about this."

Macy nodded. "Now all we need is a connection to the therapist's murder." He laughed at first, but when he met his partner's eyes, he lost the smile. He knew they both wondered if they stumbled onto something big.

Stokes turned to Macy, but did not speak. Macy liked that about Stokes, a colleague smart enough to allow him to follow that inner journey that had led to the solutions of many of their cases over their time as partners. Macy turned his thoughts back to Fleur. Could it be another coincidence that Fleur's car had been found close to Dr. Davide's house? She had followed someone and had decided to spy on him or her. Otherwise, she would not have concealed her car. She sneaked up to a house, looked inside a window or door, maybe took a picture or two.

"Stokes, did anyone find Fleur's cell phone?"

"Nothing in the report. When they found her, she had only the clothes on her back. No purse. No phone."

Macy turned to the assistant, "Find out who the carrier is, and see if we can locate the phone with its GPS. If she tossed her phone on purpose or just dropped it, its location might lead us to some clue about where she took the beating." Macy turned back to Stokes without waiting for an answer. "I want to know more about Ms. Campbell. She had phony smeared all over her. I want to know anything we can use to determine if Dr. Marsdon is the actual lover. It goes against human nature that she would direct suspicion at him when she hadn't known we were interested in him as a suspect. Heck, we had no leads on the case. Then, just for kicks, I want a background check of Marsdon's partner, Davide."

Stokes leaned over to their assistant. "Do me a favor, too. Get a photo of Dr. Davide and add him and Ms. Campbell to the search of anyone around the airport parking garage before and after the murder."

"Here's a photo from their website," the assistant said. "Easy."

"Well," Stokes said. "He looks like a slick bastard. Too pretty for his own good. Used to getting whatever he wants, I'd say. Just the type a woman would lie, cheat, and steal for."

"Maybe even murder for," Macy said.

Tate welcomed the invitation from Erin to meet for lunch. When he heard the tension in her voice, he assumed she had experienced a wave of mourning as he did off and on. Those sheets of sadness, denial, anger, but no sign of acceptance in sight. His own experience dealing with Henry Vine's death taught him that no amount of talking about those emotions made a difference. He had to let them have their way with him. He had to experience the pain and loss as part of the process no matter what the so-called experts recommended. Even if he were not a physician, he did not prescribe to the theory that mourning had a time limit that should be squelched by a pill if a patient exceeded their due-by date for complete recovery.

"I'm glad you had the free time to meet me for lunch," Erin said. She stood up to embrace him, and he reciprocated with a light kiss on her cheek.

"Any time for you," he said. He noted a hesitation in her manner that was unlike her. "Is something wrong?"

"Not wrong, necessarily."

"Yes?"

"I saw Imogen today."

Hearing her name fell on his ears like weights. "Okay."

"She wants you to visit her. I know what you're thinking," she said, holding up her hand to stop his comments. "I understand this is unfair of me to ask. I wouldn't ask if I didn't feel it's important for her but for you too. Her memories are returning more quickly than the doctor expected. She's almost there."

"What can I do? Give her absolution?"

"Now you're being facetious."

"After that night at her house, I doubt I can sit in the same room with her. I can't forget the image of Henry on that bed while she confessed how she killed him with no more emotion than she would describe her stew recipe."

"The problem is it's like she has some blockage that she believes is related to you. You were close up until this happened."

"But she killed Henry."

"What if she didn't?"

Tate looked at Erin. She looked soft, but her words sounded sharp and pointed. "What? She confessed, didn't she?"

"Yes, she confessed. I can't argue with that. You can't argue that she hasn't suffered a break with reality either. That condition can be attributed to emotional trauma and not to committing a violent act. If she's guilty, I want to get her the best sentence possible. If she's not guilty and has had this breakdown because she witnessed the crime, I want to keep her from being punished for a crime she didn't commit."

Tate leaned back in his chair. Their eyes locked—both challenging the other. "You're wrong,"

"I can see in your expression you believe this is possible. Won't you speak to her? If there's the slightest chance, Henry would want that."

"Don't try those manipulative courtroom tactics on me that you use on witnesses. I'll go meet her, but don't expect me to subscribe to your theories without someone providing tangible proof to the contrary."

Erin let out a sigh and smiled at him, but Tate ignored her.

Tate did not have cause to visit the psychiatric hospital in his specialty. He recalled comments from other medical professionals who found out early in their careers that they had no patience or tolerance required to be effective in working with the individuals with mental health issues. He understood that as he walked through the ward. An icy sterility permeated the walls, furnishings, and equipment, all the way down to the plastic-gloved hands of the nurses passing out medications. He shivered. He recalled a woman he dated once who said mental illness frightened her. He had listened with an unsympathetic ear. He considered her comment childish and insensitive and told her so. Later, he regretted his harshness. Hers had been an immature expression of an intangible fear of unpredictable behavior, the very anxiety he experienced now.

After checking in, a nurse led him to the waiting room. His stomach fluttered. Was he afraid? How should he respond to her?

He turned around to see her walking into the room. She looked frail, weak, and cautious. They both found eye contact difficult, so each looked past one another during a strained hug.

"Thank you for coming, Tate. I know you must hate me right now," Imogen said.

He saw her holding back tears and hoped to God that she kept that under control.

"Are you being treated well here?"

"They're all very kind." She paused, looking out of the window. "I know this must be hard for you to come here like this. I know Henry loved you like a son as much as you loved him like a father."

Tate could not speak. His senses overtaken by the antiseptic rooms and his grief froze him. The tightness in his throat would have prevented him from speaking if he had a response.

"I wanted to see you because my memories are coming back more every day. I haven't remembered everything yet, but I know something is wrong, and it involves you."

"Me?"

"I'm scared for you. I wish I could remember. Dr. Davenport said the memories would return more quickly if I stopped straining. After yesterday, when I had started to feel hopeful and more at peace, seeing Frankie out in the parking lot arguing with that man, well, it started something in my head that I can't explain."

"Frankie was here to see you?"

"No, I'm not allowed visits yet. I stayed here in this room after Erin left. That's when I started to people watch out this window. I didn't recognize her at first until she turned her face upward to finger-comb her hair. That's when I recognized her."

"Who was the man?"

"I don't want to cause trouble if I'm wrong."

"Just tell me who you think he is."

"Your partner, Derren Davide."

Tate opened his mouth to speak, but had no idea what to say. Being in this place must have its effects on him. A brief disorienting sensation took over. He had to think.

"Have they been seeing each other long?"

"I can't remember. If it weren't for seeing them down there, I might not have recalled their relationship at all. I wanted to see you because ever since I saw them, I've had the worst feeling that I know something bad is going to happen, but I can't bring it to the surface. Dr. Davenport said seeing you might trigger a memory."

"Has it?"

"The only bit that comes back has to do with a girl. I get flashes about her parents and friends needing closure."

"That means nothing to me," Tate said.

"I'm sorry."

"If nothing else, I've learned something I didn't know before. Not that Derren has to answer to me about his romantic affairs, but I would expect a mention."

"You don't see couples fighting the way they were who haven't been together for a while."

"I appreciate this information, Imogen. I don't know what it means yet, but it might make more sense in another context." This new information had thrown him so far afield of Henry's murder that he forgot to be angry with Imogen. "I need to go to check on some things in the office."

Neither had bothered to sit down when he arrived, so he reached over to hug her and headed toward the door. Before he turned the knob to go, he turned around.

"Thank you. Erin has the idea that you might not have killed Henry. I hope she's right."

He saw tears welling up, and left before she could say anything else.

By the time he reached his car, he had run various scenarios in his mind to pull this knowledge into what he already knew. He had to be honest that he could understand Derren keeping a relationship with one of his patients secret. Whether justified or not, plastic surgeons had the notorious reputation for bedding all their attractive patients. But that did not explain Frankie's office visits inquiring about procedures Derren could have explained to her. It also did not explain what she searched for in his office. If he and Derren worked the same days, the situation might be different. If that were the case, he might believe that she wanted to make Derren jealous.

And what about this girl Imogen spoke of? That worried him more than Derren and Frankie's relationship. Whether she realized it or not, Imogen spoke as if the girl were dead. Could this be a patient that died recently? Trauma patients did not always survive the initial physical damage, even after multiple, successful surgeries by a team of surgeons. He would check on his trauma patients in the last six months to find out if a young woman had died. Maybe the family believed one of the doctors was to blame for the death. Grief and anger at losing someone could be a volatile combination.

Session Six

Imogen saw Henry in the backyard when she came into the kitchen. Just as he had done the last six weeks, he had made her a beautiful breakfast, the cut flowers from the garden, her best cloth napkins. The smell of coffee that she could no longer drink wafted in the air, following

Henry to the porch. He started up this new ritual due to her diet restrictions of no caffeine. Imogen thought he had to be the sweetest man she had ever known. That said something considering the running around she did before she met Henry.

"Hey, honeybunch. Good morning," she said, sticking her head out the back door.

"Don't holler out that corny nickname like that. Someone might hear you. And morning to you, Granma."

He set aside the rake to join her while she ate. "How are you feeling? You look refreshed this morning, not so faint."

"I didn't need to take the pain meds last night or this morning."

"You look great, but don't overdo it, as you're prone to do."

"I won't. I haven't any plans, so I think I'll stick around here. Do some reading and catch up on my shows."

"Good. I'll be in the backyard. I'm using the hula hoe to get those weeds out of the rocks before we lose the battle. By the way, don't get worried if you notice my car's gone. I took it in for an overhaul, belts, hoses, timing chain, and the works. We can get more miles out of it before we replace it."

"Okay. I'll be here, keeping the home fires burning while my hero makes his mark on the world."

"You're kind of nuts, aren't you?" Henry said. He had started to rise from his chair, when she pulled him down.

"You wouldn't have me any other way." Imogen gave him a deep-tongued kiss before letting him up from the chair.

Dr. Davenport looked up when she stopped talking.

"Anything wrong, Imogen?"

"Not really. I remembered what I thought at the moment I kissed him."

"What was that."

"I thought how lucky we were to still have each other after his accident and my cancer."

"You haven't mentioned this before. Would you like to tell me about Henry's accident?"

"Yes, I think I would. I lived through it but I never talked about it."

Session Six continued

Imogen walked up to Henry's bed. *No matter what he looks like, act normal.* At first, his injuries were not obvious. As she came closer, she realized his worst injuries were on his left side. The police said the force of the impact when the tow truck skidded and its trailer jackknifed had caught the back of the driver's side of Henry's pickup and propelled him into the intersection. He must have had his head turned at the time of the accident. The police said a semi could not stop in time to avoid the collision, skidded and Henry drove under its trailer before he could regain control of his vehicle. Everyone she spoke to thought Henry survived by a miracle.

When she saw his injuries, she prayed for him to die. She could not see any medical treatment that could restore his face. He would be deformed the rest of his life, hiding from people, living as a hermit, crippled and hideous. Their Camelot gone.

The first time she saw Dr. Tate Marsdon, she had dismissed him as just one of the many doctors coming and going in Henry's room, or one the various nurses checking his vitals, replenishing his intravenous fluids, and determining if he was conscious. She had not slept in over twenty hours, determined not to leave Henry in what time he had left.

"Mrs. Vine? I'm Dr. Marsdon. I'll be performing surgery on your husband as soon as we run a few tests."

"Surgery?"

"I'll be performing the reconstruction to his face."

Imogen started to cry.

"Mrs. Vine, are you alright?"

"You can fix this? I had no idea."

"I'm going to do everything in my power. He's had extensive damage to the nerves and muscles in his face, but I've seen the X-rays, and believe I can restore his face."

"The other doctors told me about his head and chest injuries and how they were able to stop the bleeding. I thought that was all they could do."

"Sometimes, that's only the beginning. The primary goal is to stabilize the patient, stop bleeding, and repair internal injuries. In this case, your husband's life-threatening injuries had to be addressed first."

Imogen kissed Henry's hand. An emotional surge of tears dropped onto his hand and ran around his wrist to the sheet beneath. Someone took her by the shoulders to guide her out through the door. She leaned against the wall in the corridor to watch while prim efficiency prepared him for surgery.

Dr. Davenport studied Imogen's face when she stopped speaking. "A very emotional time for you."

"I thought it was all over for us. The end of Camelot. We were so grateful to Dr. Marsdon for giving us a second chance, not only for Henry, but for me, too. I've told him many times that words can't express how we feel about him."

Dr. Davenport smiled. "He sounds like quite a doctor. I can't wait to meet him. So, was it after Henry's surgery, he became a personal friend?"

"It started when we invited him over for dinner to thank him. We're old-fashioned like that. He and Henry hit it off right away. Our children live back east, and I guess we both missed having them around. Tate's on his own here too. We both enjoyed his company, but Henry and Tate filled a void for the other."

Imogen looked beyond Davenport. Her eyes went blurry, reliving a happy memory.

"Were you around when he met Erin?"

Imogen looked at him and grinned. "I'm responsible for that. It's a great story."

"I want to hear about that, but let's save that for tomorrow morning."

"Afraid of those feminine tears, doc?"

Imogen walked back to her room, arms clinched around her shoulders embracing her memories while trying to block out the reality.

CHAPTER SIXTEEN

Imogen leaned back on the chaise next to Dr. Davenport. She smiled back at him.

"Yes, I remember when Tate met Erin. I had a scheme up my sleeve and it worked.

"Judging from your expression, you enjoyed that evening," Davenport said.

"I did. One of the most satisfying, as matchmaking goes. Mostly because Henry didn't know and didn't have time to stop me." Imogen looked away from him and closed her eyes.

Session Seven

Imogen looked at Henry when Tate Marsdon entered the restaurant. "On his own again," she said.

Henry gave her a warning look. "*Occupe-toi tes oignons.*"

"I am minding my own business. It's just that I wish he would meet a nice girl."

"Maybe he's interested in his work right now. Don't start interfering, or I'll tell him you're up to no good."

"You wouldn't."

"I would, so stop acting like an old lady."

Imogen blew out a heavy sigh and sipped her Chardonnay while she watched Tate cross the dining room once he spotted them. When Tate arrived at their table, Henry stood to shake hands. Imogen half stood to accept a kiss on her cheek.

"Great you could join us. Busy day?"

"Not too bad. No surgeries. I haven't recovered from the eight-hour surgery on a trauma patient two nights ago."

"I don't know how you keep the pace. You can have a drink? Not on call?"

He looked down at his watch, "Not as of two hours ago."

The waiter arrived for his drink order. "Chivas."

"Thank you, sir."

"Hey, you two. Look who just walked in," Imogen said. "It's Trish DeVane. Remember last year when she stood trial for murdering her husband?"

Tate and Henry turned to watch the striking woman at the center of the scandal for three months before the jury acquitted her.

"Vogue on the outside. Vague on the inside," Henry snorted. "But just smart enough to get away with murder."

"I thought she'd left town," Tate said. "The media crucified her. I heard she couldn't leave her house without a body guard between the press and hordes of protestors at her front gate."

"She got off on a technicality," Henry said. "It was obvious she did it, but she had a good attorney."

"Who's that woman with her," Tate said.

"The star attorney herself," Henry said. "The photos in the paper didn't do her justice."

"Erin Fitzgerald. They call her the real-life Perry Mason," Imogen said. "I met her at a fundraiser a few months ago. Want to meet her?"

"Yes, she sounds interesting," Tate said, still watching the two women moving through the dining room in their direction.

Imogen walked toward the two women, said a few words, and then led them toward their table. Imogen avoided Henry's eyes, pleased to see the subdued excitement on Tate's face when they approached. "I invited them to join us," Imogen said, beaming with the self-satisfying expression she knew Henry observed.

Henry and Tate stood when the women reached the table.

"Trish and Erin, this is Tate Marsdon, *MD*," Imogen said. "Very dedicated and single plastic surgeon. Around our house, he's known as the Lord of Plastic Surgery."

"There's no need for introduction." Erin extended her hand to Tate. "I've heard of your work from Judge Bellows."

"Imogen was just telling us about *your* impressive reputation," Tate said.

Erin smiled at him, taking a seat next to Trish. Imogen caught Erin's fleeting blush under Tate's stare.

"The rest of us are still here," Trish said. Imogen noted her abrasive nature, a contrast to her soft appearance.

"My fault," Tate said. "I'm pleased to meet you both."

"I'm sure I don't need an introduction either," Trish said. "Unfortunately. Thanks for inviting us over. I don't get many social invitations these days."

"The ordeal must have been horrible for you," Imogen said.

"Well, what can one do? I'm grateful to have found Erin. I don't know where I would be now without her." Trish turned to Erin. "This is a special person. The first time I saw her, I thought someone played a joke on me by sending me a model instead of an attorney. Defense attorney Barbie I called her, hey, Erin?"

Erin blushed. "I think you're exaggerating. However, being a woman, I've had to prove myself more often in spite of my credentials. Certainly much more than a man in the same position, but I don't regret my choices. The law is a passion with me, as is defending victims of circumstantial evidence."

"Let's not talk shop this evening," Imogen said. "What do you do for relaxation, Erin?"

"I like to play tennis, but I haven't the time to join a club to find a partner. My schedule is too erratic. What I need to do is take lessons," Erin said. "Same reason I don't golf."

"I can give you tennis lessons," Tate said.

Erin gave him a skeptical look. "Are you a good player?"

"I'm very good."

"Then forget it."

"Why?"

"When I play tennis with a friend or acquaintance who's very good, I watch their frustration at my awkward playing turn into complete aggravation. Before you know it, I'm angry and hurt at their lack of patience. I decided I need a professional coach. When I have the time, I'll do it."

"I'm patient and tolerant of the inept. I don't get frustrated. I look at it more as a personal challenge. Give me a chance. I can be a good teacher."

Imogen struggled to keep her mouth closed. Her eyes switched between the two, thinking what a handsome couple they made. The modern day power couple and she would take credit for bringing them together. "Go on, Erin."

Erin grinned into a wide smile, showing off her bright green eyes against the dark red hair and creamy skin tones. "Okay."

When she finished talking, she noticed Dr. Davenport smiling back at her.

"I'm pleased with your progress. You're stronger every time I see you."

"Do you think I'll have all my memories back soon? I'm still so lost."

"Don't be impatient. Allow your thoughts to come out naturally, and don't be frustrated with yourself. The truth is not far off."

Tate and Erin settled in across from the Bellows in front of their fireplace that evening, sipping coffee after dessert. This had been their first night out since the murders. Tate went into the relaxed state that comes after a great shock has worn off. The discussions ranged from the latest surgical techniques to the Bellows' plan to install a sauna in their guesthouse. The soothing atmosphere had a hypnotic effect, pulling him deeper into restfulness.

"I still say it's a shame about Jenny Marcus," Barry said. "Beautiful girl, bright, ambitious. Probably would have made a terrible wife, though."

"Barry! What a chauvinistic comment," Lorraine said. "What's that got to do with anything anyway?"

"Not chauvinistic, dear. Think of the length of time to study to be a doctor, to establish a practice, and then build a reputation. Not much time for lollygagging around with a husband in tow. Men need attention—a lot of it, at least, according to you. I'm lucky you let me become a judge."

Lorraine rolled her eyes at him. "Anyway, I haven't seen an update in the paper on the case in the last two days. I feel bad for her parents. What a tragedy, and then not to know why she was killed. Her family must be tormented."

Tate perked up at the similarity with Imogen's comments about the girl.

"The last I read, they were checking video surveillance and asking for anyone to come forward who was at the airport in Terminal Four around that time." Erin said.

"We should talk to the police, dear," Lorraine said. "We were there. So were you, Tate. Remember?"

"I remember the flight, but I don't remember anything out of the ordinary happening that day," Tate said. Maybe Imogen's words haunted him, but he started to experience the anxiety she described when she said he was in danger.

"Did you see your partner, Derren, there?" Lorraine said. "He passed us a few minutes before we saw you, but he rushed by and didn't notice us."

"What a coincidence," Erin said. "The four of you were there at the same time on different flights." Erin looked over to Tate, who looked deep in concentration. "Is something wrong? You look funny."

"You mean like a clown?" Tate said. He would tell her about this on the way home.

"Yeah, now that you mention it," Erin said.

"I know what you mean," Barry said. "About the coincidence. How often do you run into someone you know at the airport?"

"Well, I think plenty of people saw something," Lorraine said.

"Yes, but do they realize what they saw?" Barry said. "When I hear testimony in court, so many witnesses recall events through an emotional retro-vision—describing something that turned out to be significant, but at the time they didn't give it much importance. Then, with so many travelers coming and going from other places, who is to say they've forgotten all about it because the story isn't airing in their part of the world?"

"You're right," Erin said. "Then you get the witnesses that wish they'd seen something, so they strain to go back with their retro-vision and manipulate their memories to fit the case."

"The police might never find out who did this killing," Barry said. "It happens."

Tate buckled in and turned on the car. He looked over to Erin. She had the dreamy look of someone who'd had a good time. He hated to ruin the pleasant evening, but he had to tell her. "You know I went to see Imogen today?"

"Of course. I haven't had the opportunity to ask you how it went."

"I think I get why you think she might not be guilty."

"Really? Tell me."

"I guess it's more that she wanted to talk to me to warn me of an unknown threat. I expected begging for forgiveness, please understand, that kind of bullshit. Instead, she told me how she'd seen Frankie having a fight with Derren in the parking lot outside of the room where we met—the same room where she met you."

Erin blew out a whistle. "You don't say? Anything else?"

"She talked about a girl she couldn't remember, and how she felt bad for her friends and parents. That talk gave me the creeps, but I had no idea what she meant.

That is not until the Judge and Lorraine started to talk about Jenny Marcus. They used practically the same words."

"This might be a break. Do you realize the significance of seeing Frankie and triggering that memory?"

"I avoid psychiatry as much as possible, so no. You tell me."

"This is speculation, but it could be possible that Derren was Jenny's mentor. You once said Frankie and Imogen were close. What if Frankie told her about that? Even if Derren didn't kill her, he might have been with her in the parking garage that day. What if Frankie told Imogen something incriminating, and now that Imogen has impaired memory, the details might come out during therapy. This is important. I know it."

"But what could this have to do with killing Henry?"

"I don't know yet, but I'm calling Detective Macy in the morning. I've heard they believe identifying the mentor is key."

Tate did not speak right away. When he did, his voice came out in a thunderous tone. "I knew Derren had to be a scumbag. I'm convinced he's stealing from me, but I never thought he had the capacity for this level of deviousness. I honestly don't care if he's screwing around with Frankie, so why should either of them keep that from me? But the idea he might have information about that poor murdered girl and continues to keep that a secret makes me wonder what else he's capable of doing."

CHAPTER SEVENTEEN

Detective Macy had a frustrating morning. He kept learning fragments of information in his cases, but never anything to identify the killers. He and Stokes decided to look through the evidence collected so far for anything they might have missed. The furthest he had come on the Jenny Marcus case lead him to unlikely suspects and a suspicious informant. Based on Ms. Campbell's information, he had to question Dr. Marsdon. Whether his gut told him her story felt wrong or not, he had to follow through.

Then, someone attacked Fleur while she was following Frankie. That made the idea that Frankie lied when she came here more plausible. What could this woman have to hide? She inserted herself into two of his investigations. "It's time we looked more into this Frankie Campbell. She smells worse all the time."

Stokes, who had been rolling similar ideas in his head, said, "I agree. I'd like to know her game."

At that moment, a technician rushed up to Macy's desk. "We've located Fleur Sander's phone. The address is 4263 Durango Lane. That's the next street over from where we found her car."

"You checked on who lives there?" Stokes said.

"Yes, sir," the technician said, beaming from his initiative. "Dr. Derren Davide owns the property through an LLC."

Stokes and Macy exchanged satisfied looks. "Things are starting to cook," Macy said.

The ringing telephone dampened Macy's enthusiasm. He answered it with more impatience than he intended, "Detective Macy."

"Detective, this is Erin Fitzgerald. I have information I've learned from Imogen Vine. I know she's still in care, but listen before you make any judgments."

Macy sat up straighter in his chair, poised pen over paper, and said, "Go ahead."

"Since Imogen's been in custody, she's talked about how worried she is over a girl. I've asked her friends but no one seems to know what she's talking about. Dr. Marsdon went to see her yesterday on her request. She told him she worried about his safety because of the girl. She also said she felt bad for the girl's parents and friends. He didn't think much about it because he had no idea what she meant until dinner last night."

She paused. "Go ahead," he said.

"During our dinner with the Bellows, the subject came up about the Jenny Marcus murder. You know, the usual speculation and comments about her family dealing with that loss and not understanding why. Tate told me later those were almost the same words Imogen used about the girl." Erin paused to take a deep breath.

"Anything else?"

"Yes. Imogen witnessed a big fight between a man and a woman. They were in the parking lot outside of the hospital. She swears the two people were Frankie Campbell and Dr. Derren Davide. This could be a link in Imogen's mind. Her memory is returning more quickly than the doctors expected, but she's not to the point of giving evidence. However, the fact that they have had a relationship in secret might have a bearing on the Jenny

Marcus case."

"Ms. Fitzgerald. Thank you for bringing this to my attention. This information could prove to be more important than you know."

"It's not only because Imogen is my client and a close friend of Dr. Marsdon, but I'm starting to wonder if she really killed her husband. One puzzle keeps leading to another."

"Unfortunately, we still have no leads in your friend's case. We've gone through the mail your assistant provided, but nothing. The answer has to be in your current caseload. Have you any fresh perspective?"

"No, I don't. I have only the two active clients, Tim Actworth and Imogen Vine. Nothing suggests that element in either situation."

"Well, there must be something we haven't considered. Please keep that in mind. We'd like to solve Hermione's case as much as the others."

"I appreciate that, Detective. If I think of anything, I'll let you know."

"We'll follow up on the information you provided."

"Thank you. Goodbye," Erin said.

Macy had a vertigo sensation that caused him to overlap the cases. Maybe he worked too long without a break. "Guess what I just learned?"

"Well?" Stokes said.

"Our Ms. Campbell is seeing Dr. Davide. Imogen Vine saw them arguing slash fighting yesterday. Although we can't be sure she's not creating false memories, Erin said seeing them triggered a fear for Dr. Marsdon. Imogen is still talking about her worries about a girl. Erin thinks this has to do with Jenny Marcus. Until Imogen gets her memory back in working order, we can't rely on her, but we can take a new look at the situation."

Stokes went inward for a moment before speaking. "And given that she walked in here and told us bare-faced lies gives credence to a concern for Dr. Marsdon. Our Frankie laid it on heavy enough that he murdered the girl. It sounds more like Dr. Davide did the deed and she's sacrificing someone to protect her lover."

The two men traded impish grins, one of the unspoken signals between them over the years.

"Maybe we'll get lucky and solve the Jenny Marcus case," Macy said. "Let's get cell phone records for both of them. That could prove to be most interesting."

Tate had seen enough botched plastic surgery procedures that he no longer showed surprise at the lengths some plastic surgeons would go to make a quick buck. This morning, he had a routine case of a woman who had developed a severe infection from a breast augmentation performed by another surgeon she declined to identify. She had told him this doctor had dismissed her concerns, so she decided not to return to him when the infection flared up. She had learned about Tate from another patient and hoped he could solve her problem.

He had seen infections before that ranged from a minor infection treated with antibiotics to the more serious staph infection caused by exposed drain tubes or tainted bandages. He expected to open her incision, find the cause, scrape and sterilize the area and replace the existing implants to avoid recontamination.

He joined his patient in the surgery suite where Paul, the anesthesiologist, had already put her under. Rachelle had arranged for his regular scrub nurse, Trina. Lissa, his favorite circulating nurse, could not make it so he had to settle for her substitute, Nancy.

By the time he began the procedure, now routine and mechanical to him after all these years, his thoughts had moved two steps ahead. He made the incisions and took out the implants from both breasts. He looked down to decide if he had to reevaluate his initials assessment. The breasts looked unnatural and misshapen. Regardless of the condition of the breast before augmentation, removing implants returned them to a natural form, so he knew he had a problem.

He reached inside to feel around the open cavity when his gloved fingers found another implant. He repeated the action on the opposite side and found the same. He placed all four implants on a tray and examined them. Not only were they different sizes, a 400 cc and a 200 cc from each breast, but the larger implants had discolored at a faster rate. That meant one set was older. *What the heck!* He would record the four serial numbers later, but he photographed them, and set them aside to preserve as evidence.

"Doctor, what's wrong?"

"I hate to say it, but another doctor somewhere is using recycled implants. I think you know what that means. Don't discard them. I need to find out where these came from."

"What do you mean?" Nancy had turned pale and Tate thought sweaty as well.

"I mean it's suspicious that one woman has two sets of implants when we have available access to 600cc implants, but the fact that one set is older makes me wonder if the doctor buys off the black market."

"Oh," Nancy said.

"Is there a problem, Nancy?" Tate, Trina, and Paul exchanged looks.

"I remember this patient. Dr. Davide did her

augmentation at another surgery center. I assisted, but I didn't notice him using two implants on each side. I certainly didn't think the implants were used either. I don't want to get into trouble. I swear I didn't notice anything." Nancy trembled and looked ready to burst into tears.

"Pull yourself together. You're a nurse. We need to finish this procedure. We'll talk about this later," Tate said. He returned to the patient, found the source of infection—an area in both breasts where the two implants met. For the patient's sake, he controlled his rage.

After he brought the patient through surgery believing he had significantly improved her state of health and attractiveness, he took the implants and the list of serial numbers to his office and looked them up on the national breast implant registry. The list of patients receiving these implants two years apart had both died under different circumstances a week apart.

"Oh my God!" Tate's senses went into overload when he recognized a bottom feeder phenomenon called corpse harvesting.

Unlike donating a body to a medical school for scientific research or legally donating organs for transplants, these notorious cases involved employees of funeral homes and crematoriums stealing and transporting bodies to a factory-like facility where workers extracted reusable devices, everything from dental implants to bladder slings, but also blood, skin, and tendons. The multi-million dollar industry mortified the public, associating the grim practice as modern day body snatching.

To have this label attached to his own practice could ruin him. And for a patient to suspect they carried a medical device inside them that had been inside a dead person would mortify almost everyone, but a ghoul.

After all the death he had seen this week, he was in the mood to fantasize murdering Derren and claiming self-defense. He could feel his hands around Derren's neck, squeezing until he gasped his last breath.

He pulled himself out of the fantasy with deep breathing. He had to keep calm and focused, and do what it took to avert a guilt-by-association public relations nightmare. He gathered up the evidence, including a USB drive of the photos throughout the procedure, and drove them to his safe deposit box at the bank. He had started his car when he saw his office calling.

"Dr. Marsdon. This is Trina. We have another problem with your patient. She's not responding to any of the intravenous pain meds I've given her."

Tate set aside his initial impression that this had something do with Derren. But, dammit, this simple procedure had turned into something bigger. "She shouldn't have that much pain. Give her two 325 mg Percocets. I'm on my way back."

After this morning's revelation, Tate did not take anything for granted. He had not had a patient unable to respond to intravenous pain meds, except in the case of someone with a drug addiction problem who needed larger doses. This patient had no history of drug abuse. To the contrary, she listed no prescription history on her patient form. His instinct told him to check the drugs cabinet for tampering.

He rushed in to recovery. Trina stood next to the patient, holding her hand. The woman looked pale, but cheerful. He saw the relief in her expression when she saw him, the look of trust that he would make everything better. "How are you doing now?"

"Much better, doctor. I don't like to complain, but the soreness in my chest got to me."

"As long as we found a solution, that's the good part."

"So, how did the procedure go? Did you find the cause of the infection?"

Tate hesitated. Trina's eyes were on him. He couldn't lie, but he knew he could not tell her what he discovered. A sensitive woman like that would go to pieces. "Yes, I found the cause of the infection, cleaned up the area, and replaced your implants." Thank God for that, he thought.

Relieved, she leaned deeper into her pillow. He saw the drug-induced haze fogging her vision. He nodded to Trina, who continued to hold her hand.

He took the time to check out the IVs. They looked functional. He went into the locked drugs cabinet to check for tampering with the bottles of morphine. Upon close inspection, he saw tiny needle marks in the wrapping of the unopened bottles. He checked the other pain medications for tampering. Every bottle had the same markings. He knew he had better have these checked to be sure that they contained the drug on their label. He thought back to his initial impression that this also had a link to Derren. If not him, he had a second thief in the house.

CHAPTER EIGHTEEN

Frankie stopped to check if all her employees had shown up on time before leaving. She slammed the back door of her restaurant kitchen. Some days she hated her life, the pressure of running a full-service restaurant, maintaining quality, managing staff, keeping up to code, always in dread of the next new restaurant that might lure away her patrons. What made it work for her was the way she managed her money. Never running an account with the vendors by paying cash daily as they delivered supplies meant that she had a good idea of her cash position every night. Some would say she did all right, but at the end of a long day, going home to an empty, albeit luxurious home, she would tell them success was a crock.

It had occurred to her before that this dissatisfaction with her life had been the primary incentive to get involved with Derren, her plastic surgeon's partner. She often wondered what he saw in her. Sure, she was attractive in an athletic way, toned and flexible from her silky thick dark blonde hair right down to the tips of her polished toenails, but so were a thousand other women in Phoenix and Scottsdale society. The internal dialogue that went on inside her head got ugly sometimes, convinced that he had a mother complex, or that he was using her for convenient sex. The old "open-door, open-leg" policy.

Those insecurities kept resurfacing, especially when he insisted their affair be a secret from Dr. Tate and their office staff. No matter how she tried to justify his attitude, the screams continued to grow louder inside her head. She was too far gone. Attached to him now, so deeply in love with him he consumed her thoughts, controlled her behavior, and left no doubt she could not leave if her life depended on it. This reminded her of playing too close to the edge of a cliff as a child, unable to draw away from the danger.

She thought of that cliff now. She sorted through her actions the last few weeks. In particular, the night Derren called for her help. How could she have known then how ugly this situation would get?

She had gotten home late from the restaurant. In one of her banquet rooms, they had hosted a special event, a celebration or a reception, she lost track. The number of actual guests exceeded the estimates, and left her scrambling to provide the food and deliver good service without the customer knowing the state of panic they caused. Everyone went home happy, full, and loaded. By the time the restaurant closed, she could think of nothing better than to fall into bed.

She took off one shoe at a time while walking in from the garage, and looked forward to a hot bath when her cell phone rang. "Who the hell is this?" she said aloud, hearing the echo bounce off the metal and ceramic surfaces, but her innate professionalism took over before she answered. "Frankie Campbell."

"It's me," Derren said. "What are you doing?"

"I just walked in. We had a busy night. We…"

"Yeah, whatever. Listen, something's happened. I need your help."

"Sure. What?"

"Come over here."

"Now? It's after one in the morning," Frankie said. She resented the command but knew she would go.

"I wouldn't ask if it weren't important." Frankie recognized the tone that implied doing what he asked was the least she could do for him.

"I'm on my way," she said. What was it that allowed her to see what was happening, but left her powerless to stop the accelerating momentum?

When she arrived at his home, she pulled around to the back and parked in front of the garages, and walked to the back door. She looked down at her cell phone to read two fifteen. She hoped he had something more important than a booty call. She turned the doorknob and walked inside his sterile white kitchen.

He rushed in from another room and said, "What took you so long?"

"You're welcome for coming out in the middle of the night to do you a favor."

Derren squinted at her for a moment. She thought he looked as if he was holding back one of his sharp remarks. "I'm sorry. It's just that I'm in a terrible state. The most horrible thing has happened."

I'm here now, so tell me," Frankie said. She walked to the refrigerator, pulled out an opened bottle of Chardonnay, and poured a glass.

"Don't drink too much. You need a clear head."

"For what?"

"You'd better sit down." He took her hand, led her to the dining room, and pulled out a chair. "There's been a death, and I might be implicated."

"Who? Why?"

"A young med student I've been *mentoring*."

"You mean *screwing*."

He ignored her. "She met me at Sky Harbor in the parking garage close to my car to bring my keys. We were in her car when I remembered I left my glasses inside the airport. When I came back, she was dead. She looked like she'd been strangled."

"How can that be an accident?"

Derren chose his words with care. "It's not what you think. We had a disagreement. Things got heated. I guess I accidentally strangled her, though I didn't think I hurt her. She was yelling, and I just wanted her to be quiet."

Frankie leaned away from him and flicked her glass in his direction. She watched the effects of the clear liquid running down his face and onto his crisp white shirt. "You asshole! You were sleeping with her? Or were you trying to and she said, no?"

"Don't be so provincial in your thinking. We're grownups, not bound to each other by the social morays that dictate others' actions. We have a relationship that works, but that doesn't mean we cannot have more than one relationship."

"What a load of bullshit. That's your elitist speak to justify your actions. Now I know why you want our relationship secret, so you appear available to every woman you fancy."

"You make it sound sordid and common. I didn't call you over here to argue about your value system. I need you to help me get out of this mess."

"How am I supposed to do that?"

"I want you to start telling your friends that Tate's been mentoring the girl. I saw him at the parking garage the same time, so he can be implicated if everyone believes he had a relationship with her."

"What's to say this med student hasn't already told her friends you were the one, and not Dr. Tate?"

"She didn't. I made sure," Derren said, averting his eyes from hers.

"So this is your routine with women. Get them to keep the affair secret so no one finds out about the others?"

"I'm a doctor. I have to be careful of my reputation. That's the only reason."

"What difference does that make? You must think I'm stupid."

Derren reached over, lifted her from the chair, pressing her into the wall behind her. He took her mouth in his, kissing her until she was breathless. Her body gave into him, legs weakened, his body the only impetus to keep her standing. She responded by pushing her body into his. The more she responded, the gentler his kisses, then he whispered into her ear, "I don't think you're stupid. I know you're in love with me, and you'll do what I tell you to do."

Frankie knew he was right. She would do what he wanted even knowing that hurting someone else to save him was wrong. She knew she could go to jail as an accomplice, but she did not care. She did not have a choice.

Now, looking back, she saw she had so many other options. After that fight at the hospital yesterday where he more than told her he was using her, she had to fight for survival. She couldn't count on anyone for help this time. With everything she had done for him, she would not let him get away with discarding her.

CHAPTER NINETEEN

Macy and Stokes had been discussing their next move. A temporary lull in their conversation allowed the surrounding keyboard clatter to overtake the room. Fresh coffee, cheese Danish pastries, and orange juice to make the rest feel healthy sat between their adjoining desks. They reached for a pastry at the same time, making them chuckle at the synchronization that had evolved from their long years as partners.

"The way I see it," Macy said, struggling to speak through a mouthful. "We need a warrant to enter his property to search for the phone and hope he hasn't found it already. Once we have the physical proof, we can bring him in for questioning."

"Ask him about his relationship with Frankie. See if we can get him to admit he knew Jenny Marcus."

"He won't talk without a lawyer. Chances are we won't get much. He'll be too smart to say anything once he knows we're on to him."

"You're right. Damn lawyers," Stokes said. "Do we have the phone records for the three here yet?"

Macy pressed a button on his phone and waited for an answer. "How're we coming with background checks we requested? Have the cell phone companies gotten back to us yet?"

A male voice on the other end, hasty and tinny, said, "Just in. Be right up."

"Right. I have a little idea. Let's use the CCTV footage from the areas around Jenny Marcus's condo, the airport parking garage, Frankie's restaurant, Erin Fitzgerald's condo, and around Dr. Davide's home. Run photos of everyone involved in these cases. And one last area— Delia's office. I have a *hunch*."

"Interesting segue," Stokes said. "Are you reaching, or do you know something you haven't let me in on?"

"It bugs me. That's all. Except for the Delia case, there are too many cross-wires for everything to be a coincidence. Imogen Vine kills Henry Vine. Her lawyer's friend is murdered. Erin Fitzgerald is dating Dr. Marsdon, whose partner turns out to be messing around with Frankie, a good friend of Imogen Vine. Someone attacks Fleur when she follows Frankie to Derren's home. Frankie tries to implicate Dr. Marsdon in Jenny Marcus's murder. How much more twisted can this get?"

Stokes stared down at his Danish, and then looked over to Macy. "When you spit it out like that, you're right."

"And," Macy said. "How much farther do we need to go to connect the Delia murder? Her daughter sent over the missing patient file. I think we should look at that with a fresh eye. Could this be Frankie using an alias? I can't see Tim Actworth being so dumb that he would murder his therapist then take another patient's file with him."

"Yes, did Detra say the file described an older woman having an affair with a younger man?"

"Sure did. Now that we know about this affair Frankie and Derren have been having, that fits."

"But what's the motive for all this killing?" Stokes leaned back, arms stretched, head resting in his hands. "A case of one murder covers another. Reacting on the no-turning-back-now attitude?"

"More than likely. None of these people are professional criminals. Whoever is doing this is acting impetuously. Striking out as the situation arises. That makes whoever it is vulnerable to mistakes. That's when we catch him or her."

Macy called the technician he had spoken to before to revise his instructions. He listened for several seconds, and turned to Stokes, "Warrant's in. Let's go."

Tate anticipated confronting Derren that day. Even when he had no appointments, Derren seemed to show up and hang out in his office. Today of all days, he did not call in or show up. Tate did not think that Derren knew he had been found out, but there he sat, waiting to pummel the guy, his anger barometer rising without the relief that would come with spewing his anger toward the source of his rage.

"Right," Tate said. He had not noticed he spoke until his voice got his attention. He flushed at that loss of control. He needed to get this sorted tonight. His nerves could not stand the idea of holding this in until tomorrow. *The jerk is probably home sucking up the drugs he stole.* He would take a drive over there. He did not need witnesses to hear Derren confess. The evidence spoke for him.

He packed up his office, locked his safe and his office door, and headed up to Durango Hills. His hands had not stopped shaking during the hours he waited at the office for Derren. Adding to that now, his hands sweated on the steering wheel—an uncomfortable slippery sensation. The closer he came to Derren's neighborhood, the harder his chest pounded. Adrenalin.

When he drove onto Durango Drive, he intended to pull into Derren's driveway until he saw several serious sedans parked there and in front of the property. Curiosity got the better of him, so he pulled over and got out. He stood as an observer for several minutes until two men he recognized came toward him.

"Dr. Marsdon. Good to see you," Macy said, extending his hand.

"Looks like trouble here," Tate said, shaking Stokes hand. "Is Derren home?"

"No, he isn't. And we have several questions we'd like him to answer." Macy turned to point at an officer carrying a plastic bag with a phone inside. "We found Fleur's cell phone around the side of his house."

Tate felt light-headed. Too much anger, too little food. Now shock added to that cocktail. He reeled back against his car door as a prop until he oriented himself. "You're saying Derren attacked Fleur. On top of what I've discovered today, I could kill him right now."

"No need to go to those extremes," Stokes said. "Let us take care of Dr. Derren Davide. Beating a slip of a girl half to death, even the guys inside have a code."

Tate had not meant to show it, but a smile slipped out at the thought.

"What did you mean when you said, 'what I've discovered today?'" Stokes leaned in conspiratorially.

"I intended to report this first to the medical board. However, under the circumstances, I feel it's just as appropriate to tell you. It might have some relevance."

"We'd appreciate whatever you can tell us," Macy said.

"I kept evidence of harvested implants that I removed from one of his former patients this morning. I also discovered something irregular with the intravenous pain medications. I've had the medication sent out for testing, so I have no absolute proof. I suspect that he's substituted these Class A narcotics with something less potent. The same patient this morning had no pain relief until we gave her tablets."

"When do you expect those results back?" Macy's eyes glistened in his excitement.

"I told them to rush, so I expect tomorrow. It's a simple test to verify the drugs, unlike trying to verify an unidentified substance against thousands."

"This goes to motivation," Macy said to Stokes.

Tate looked confused. "What do you mean?"

Stokes took the lead, "We wondered why he and Frankie are trying to pin a murder on you. I only tell you because we thought it suspicious. Frankie came down to our office to tell us all about the affair you were having with Jenny Marcus. This new scenario makes much more sense when you consider what Derren has to lose professionally. His type would always think if they could get rid of one person, no one would find out what he'd been up to."

Tate could not think of anything to say.

"We hadn't called you in for an interview yet, although we're ready to do that. None of what we had made sense before. I'd like you to bring down your evidence and the result of the medication testing and make a formal statement. One more thing."

"Yes?" Tate said, grateful he could speak again.

"Don't confront him on your own. Leave this to us."

Tate nodded. He agreed happily. Physical confrontation was not his forte, although he was sure he could beat the crap out of Derren with little effort.

"If you hear from him, let one of us know," Macy said, handing two cards to Tate.

"Right."

"I think it's best you went home now. We have the forensics folks here doing their jobs and officers available if he comes home. And if he sees you here, knowing you have an ongoing disagreement, he's likely to think you're involved with what's going on here."

"Glad to go. I'll see you downtown in the morning."

Tate went to his car, backed out, and then passed the crew of police on his way down the hill. He had the sadistic satisfaction that Derren's life as he knew it was practically over. The best revenge is when you let the other person do himself in. There would be no blood on his hands."

Derren reclined the passenger seat and stretched out. He legs did not extend all the way, but that was the least of his problems. When his neighbors called him, one after another, to tell him the police were all over his property, he panicked and drove to Parker without stopping. His head swirled with visions of prison—those meaty brutes violating him physically or mentally, or both. Going to prison meant something worse than a death sentence. Until he figured a way out of this mess, he had to stay hidden.

He cowered from the cover of the *Arizona Republic* newspaper racked in the hotel lobby, afraid to see his picture splashed on the front page with a subtitle like, "Wanted. Dead or Alive." He half expected a cautious welcome from the hotel clerk who, he believed, pressed a silent signal alarm to the police. Instead, she gave him the smile he expected from women, the flirtatious warmth exuding hope and availability.

Modern technology made it difficult to remain anonymous for long, but he found cash in advance to be an incentive. He checked into the Parker Motel under a false name and walked the stairs to his apartment suite.

His burner phone rang. Frankie's number popped up, but he decided not to answer and wait to hear what she had to say in her message. The notification beeped. *Okay. Let's hear what she has to say.*

"Derren, where are you? I went by your house, but I saw cops everywhere. What does it all mean? Please call me. What's going on?"

He cringed. This inexpressible resistance to her came slowly, the indefinable sense that he could not trust her. He had shrugged it off at first, blaming himself for asking her to help him out of the jam. What had he been thinking?

He thought about Jenny and that last time with her in the car. Sure, he hit her, but he did not believe the force he used could have killed her. Yet, minutes later between when he left and returned, she had died. Anyone with anything to lose would have reacted as he did. He made a mistake asking for help from a person who expected him to pay with gratitude and servitude the rest of his life.

Was that the source of the anxiety he experienced when he thought of Frankie? He unlocked the door of his suite. As he crossed the threshold, he wondered if he fled to Parker to escape the police or her.

CHAPTER TWENTY

Tate saw Detective Macy's notepad with a bulleted list scrawled in an abbreviated handwriting style. He had second thoughts about this interview, especially without legal counsel, but he had decided yesterday that the cops needed what he knew to reinforce their case against Derren. He still seethed every time he thought about his patient yesterday.

"Thanks for taking the time to come down," Macy said. When Tate did not answer, he looked down at his notes. "I'm going to ask you some questions that might be offensive. Don't take it that way. For the sake of following every lead to a satisfactory end, we have to ask the uncomfortable questions. Most people involved in these circumstances don't volunteer what they know without prodding. I appreciate the fact that you're here voluntarily without an attorney. You can terminate this interview at any time you feel I'm stepping across the line."

"Certainly, Detective. Ask away."

"One. Were you or did you ever have a romantic relationship with Frankie Campbell?"

Tate knew his face had gone red from the heat of the sudden enlargement of blood vessels in his cheeks. He bit hard on the inside of his cheek to stop it, but Macy had seen his reaction. "Absolutely not."

"You'll understand later, but let's get these questions

out of the way. Then I'll explain everything."

"All right. Go on."

"Two. Were you at any time a mentor for Jenny Marcus?"

"The murdered medical student at the airport? No. I haven't participated in the program for over a year."

"Three. Have you had personal conversations with Frankie Campbell concerning a relationship with Jenny Marcus?"

Tate scoffed. "Seriously?" To Macy's nod, he said, "Again, absolutely not."

"Frankie Campbell came in here the other day and made these statements. She said she feared you had killed Jenny and thought we should know."

Tate's head started spinning, the room dreamlike and distorted. Reality grew twisted and dark. "I'd say she's protecting Derren. Yesterday, I learned that Derren is the man she's seeing."

"Right," Macy said. "Deflect blame from him and onto you."

"I'm starting to wonder if there's a decent bone in his body."

"This is speculation without solid evidence. We have both of you entering the parking garage at Sky Harbor, but no proof against him or you that either of you went near Jenny Marcus. However, we do know that Fleur followed Frankie to Derren's home. We found her car concealed three houses down and her cell phone on his property. I see every likelihood that one or both of them assaulted Fleur when they caught her spying."

"So that's what went on yesterday," Tate said. He relaxed.

"Why were you there yesterday?"

"To confront Derren about his medical practices."

"Let's go over everything you told me yesterday. For the record." Macy took up his pencil and flipped his pad to a fresh page.

"I'll give you the morbid first. He's corpse harvesting breast implants. Buying them used on the black market. That's based on implants I removed from a patient. I didn't learn she had been one of his patients at a different clinic. My nurse told me. I only put the facts together. That's not a great leap. Other cases have surfaced, one in New York, another in Texas."

Tate saw Macy's face drain of color, and wanted to laugh at his incredulous expression, so much like his a few minutes ago.

"Anything else relevant?"

Tate felt his anger return with thoughts of the stolen drugs and his patient suffering needlessly. "I suspect he's been substituting the narcotics in the office for something else, maybe saline. The test results haven't come back. In one case, you have unethical practices and the other outright criminal behavior. I was furious enough to kill him when all this came to light yesterday morning."

"Do you think he has a drug problem?"

"He doesn't exhibit the usual signs," Tate said. "But I'd prefer he had an addiction than to know it's all about greed."

"We've been unable to locate him. Any ideas about where we might look?"

"We've never had that kind of relationship. We'd discuss practice-related matters. That's about the extent of it."

Macy took a dismissive attitude, and Tate knew the information sharing period had ended. "Thanks for coming down here. I'm sorry about those questions, but we had to ask for the record."

"I understand," Tate said, standing up. "Did Erin Fitzgerald contact you about Imogen's memories?"

"Yes, she did. but I already had my doubts that what Ms. Campbell told us held much merit."

"All the times you think you're in control. When I look back to the extensive background check on Derren, I'm surprised how easily he deceived me."

"We see it every day, Doctor. Those types keep us in business," Macy said. He started to rise and said, "Thanks again for coming in. I'd appreciate a heads up when the drug analysis comes in."

Tate walked out of police headquarters disoriented, unsteady, expecting the sidewalk to undulate and throw him off balance. He had not seen or heard the last of his problems with Derren, but he had the worst behind him—discovery.

"It's time to bring Ms. Campbell in for a little chat. She has a lot to answer for." Stokes walked in and sat at his desk, facing Macy.

"I agree. She should be at her restaurant now. Let's give her a surprise visit."

The same technician rushed up to their desks, breathless and excited. "I have the results we've been waiting for."

"Sit down," Macy said. "Breathe and tell us about it."

"First, we scanned the footage from the airport and found both Davide and Marsdon going into the parking garage within fifteen minutes of each other. Funny thing is we saw Davide leave and return after that. Remember expanding the search on the traffic CCTVs? Well, we found the same car around in all five incidents. It's registered to Dr. Davide."

"Let's be clear," Macy said. "CCTV also caught his vehicle at Delia Ferguson's office, Erin Fitzgerald's condo, the medical building where Fleur Sanders was left for dead, and Imogen Vine's house the day we established Henry Vine died?"

"Yes, sir," the technician said, still gulping air. "I have the background checks on Frankie Campbell and Derren Davide. Nothing much on her, but he has a long list of financial problems that's been following him the last ten years. Somehow, he's able to pull himself out of trouble at the last minute."

Macy stroked an imaginary goatee and looked into the distance. "We have enough to bring him in. I'm going to enjoy this interview."

Derren looked down at his ringing burner phone. The familiar caller did not ring him unless he had a problem. Fear ripped through his midsection. He fought back the inclination to ignore the call—the basic instinct of survival, he guessed.

"Yeah," Derren said.

"What are you playing at?"

"What do you mean?"

"The package you left at the hospital. What's the idea of leaving Valium suppositories? Is that your idea of a joke?"

"No, that's not what I put in the package. I put four boxes of medical grade cocaine. I swear." Sweat poured from his brow. His hands trembled. "Someone must've seen me and replaced it with the Valium."

"I don't care how it happened. I want what I paid for. You get it to me by the end of the day. Period. I don't have to tell you the consequences of trying to rip me off if you don't."

"I'm not in Phoenix. How can I…"

"I'm not interested in excuses. Make it happen."

Derren heard the disconnect echo in his head like clapping cymbals. His hands moist with sweat, allowed the phone to slip onto the floor. He looked down at his fingers that easily wielded a scalpel—applying his expert surgical skills in intricate procedures on children and infants. Losing that which made him unique and a standout among other surgeons terrified him. If he did not deliver as promised, they threatened to ruin his hands.

He had emptied out the office reserve of Dilaudid and medical grade cocaine. Even if he were in Phoenix, he had no street source, no emergency stash.

His only option had to be another outpatient surgery center. That meant breaking and entering. No question that he had to make the choice between jail and permanent mutilation. At least, he could perform surgeries in prison and hope to get out still young enough to practice again.

Derren looked around the room at its modest furnishings, so different from his home in Phoenix. What had his life come to that he had to run and hide like a criminal. Correction, he nodded in the mirror, he *was* a criminal. He picked up a towel, held it under cold running water, and wiped his face and neck. He ran his fingers through his thick blond hair and looked transfixed at his own reflection. "You'll get out of this."

Minutes later, he had his tablet out searching the Internet for surgery centers between Parker and Phoenix. He found a couple with limited hours that had potential. He decided on one close to Interstate 95 that took him back to Interstate 10 on his way to Phoenix. He could drop in before closing time and ask for a tour. If he were lucky, he could sneak away and hide. If he were not lucky, he would scope out the locks and windows to break in after everyone left. Once he got the drugs, he would make the delivery at the hospital and drive back to Parker. He looked around the room again reluctant to leave his temporary refuge.

Nurse Shapiro had keen senses one would expect from a diminutive bird-like creature with a narrow beak for a nose. Derren wondered if she smelled his fear, like predators do.

"I was driving back to Phoenix and wanted to get a look at your facility," Derren said.

"Well, doctor, there isn't a lot to see. We're a small facility. We mostly handle emergencies. Sometimes minor elective surgeries. The main hospital in this area is twenty miles away, so the locals prefer coming here. When we're open, that is. Our limited budget keeps our doors closed until we get an emergency call or one of the doctors requests a slot."

She leaned against the reception counter and waited. Derren felt her eyes bore into him with a skepticism and disapproval as if she read his every thought. How much easier this would have been with a young nurse easily flattered by a doctor's attention. No such luck.

"What about a quick look around as you're closing up? I'm looking for a clean environment, modern equipment, all available supplies on hand. Just because I do cosmetic procedures, I'm still particular."

"I guess it won't hurt," she said. She still looked suspicious, but cooperative. "Come this way."

Derren followed her through reception, pre-op, the surgery suite, and then to post-op recovery. He had spotted the drugs cabinet but made a point not to ask about it or appear too interested. He would not have the opportunity to hide with her leading him around. He checked the windows and doors as they walked.

Discouraged at the high quality of their sealed windows, he asked to use the restroom before heading out. He saw an opportunity in the narrow casement window. He could fit through there. He used a paper towel to release the lock and returned to Nurse Shapiro.

"Thanks for staying to show me around. I'll get out of here and let you get on with closing."

"Thank you for showing an interest in our facility. We hope to hear from you soon, doctor," she said. Her perfunctory manner, as unwelcoming as it was, showed that quality of automatic responses certain people exhibit when they're not paying attention. That worked to his advantage.

He drove a mile down the road, pulled over and parked. He sat with his hands grasping the steering wheel, wondering how much time to wait before he went back. He knew he should be hungry, but that idea nauseated him. He leaned back in his seat, closed his eyes, and breathed in the comforting smell of leather upholstery. After this, no more. He would find another way to make extra money. These people were dangerous.

The sun set behind a short mountain. Derren waited until its last glow receded and left the area outside the floodlights of the rest area dark and uninviting. He opened the car door and stood up to stretch. His hands shook—nerves for sure, but his mood lightened at the prospect of averting at least one crisis.

He got back in the car and reached to his backseat for his gym bag and pulled out a T-shirt, sweat pants, and running shoes. He quickly changed, grabbed plastic surgical gloves, and set out on foot back to the surgery center.

He walked through the desert in its natural state barely visible in front of him without a bright moon but easy to define small trees and bushes at his feet. From the edge of the parking lot, he scanned the building for signs of activity. All clear. He slipped his key inside his shoe and went into a slow run toward the back of the building.

He found the restroom window. He pulled out the plastic gloves, stretched them over his long fingers, and pulled at the edge with his fingertips. The crusty metal rim moved with his motion. It would be tight. When the window had stretched open as far as it would go, he pulled himself up and bent through the opening head first, hands on the sill for leverage. When he was thigh high into the room, he leaned forward to allow his legs inside, and jumped to the floor.

He blinked in the darkness, surprised he had not broken something on his way into this tiny space. He reached for the door handle and stopped. It occurred to him this door might be wired for security. He moved the handle in slow increments, but nothing happened.

The low lights in the hall provided enough ambient light to make his way to his destination. He tiptoed until he found the drugs cabinet. He recognized the standard lock and smiled. Just like the one at his office. He pulled his key out of his shoe and worked it into the lock until he heard it release. Amazing, he thought, how many of these locks varied little from the others, enough to use one key in place of another.

He opened the cabinet door with care and scanned its interior until he found the boxes he wanted. He let out a sigh and smiled. *How easy is this.* He slipped through the facility back to the bathroom, and out through the window.

He jogged back to his car, a weight lifted from his shoulders. The interior of his car comforted him, a haven from the vulgar outside world. He fired up its engine and moved south onto the highway to get back to the hospital, and put this part of his nightmare behind him.

Then out of the darkness behind him, he saw the flashing red lights of a police car. He had a second to decide whether to stop and give up, or to see if the money he paid for this Tesla had been worth it. He jammed the accelerator and blasted into the darkness of the highway.

His heart pounded in violent thumps. His chest on the verge of erupting from his chest. His eyes blurred from the nervous sweat moving down his forehead. Could he control the car at this speed? His moist hands gripped the steering wheel tighter to compensate for his impaired vision. He did not dare let go at this speed, but he had to wipe his eyes. If only he could escape those flashing lights. He checked his car's speed now—110 mph.

He looked up from the speedometer too late to see the semi lurching in front of him on an uphill incline. He swerved to miss the back end of the massive bumper, but hit a verge meant for runaway trucks. His car jerked him forward when it came to its abrupt stop. His head bounced off the steering wheel. Sorry he had disconnected airbag. The Tesla bounced out of a ravine and into the solid mass of a giant saguaro. The angry cactus bent over from the assault slammed down on the roof of his vehicle, pinning down the falcon wing doors and his unconscious body.

CHAPTER TWENTY ONE

Tate heard the news of Derren's accident from Rachelle when he arrived in his office. Why did he think that Derren cheated him out of a confrontation?

"So what happened," he said. He hoped he kept his indifference hidden.

"All I heard on the news this morning was the cops were chasing him south on I-95 driving over a hundred miles an hour when he hit a verge and flipped over. An ambulance rushed him to the La Paz County Hospital. No news about his condition. It's funny no one's called this morning. Do you think someone's called his family?"

"His family lives in Denmark now. They might have already been contacted."

"I took it on myself to cancel all his office appointments. I switched most of them to you. I hope you don't mind. I thought you'd want to keep them as patients here, like you do for vacations."

Tate smiled. The perfect front office personality, efficient and clever. "You did the right thing on both counts." Tate had decided before this dismal news not to mention any of what he learned to anyone else. The fewer that knew, the better.

He sat down at his desk and leaned back. The last week had been as bad as he had seen. He had little time to mourn Henry or Erin's friend, Hermione, as he thought he should. Patients turning on him and on each other, police detectives interviewing him as a murder suspect, finding out his partner was a devious dickhead who might ruin his practice—without his family around him, at least he had Erin to stabilize him.

He had an overwhelming sense of urgency that he needed to be with her. He resisted the urge to call her. He found comfort that he would see her later.

Macy gave Stokes a knowing look after the call that informed them their prime suspect in multiple murders had almost killed himself eluding the police. They chuckled when they learned the officer only wanted to alert him his lights were not turned on. The discovery of the surgery center theft came later.

"I don't know how this can get any better. It explains his erratic behavior and irrational belief he could get away with murder."

"Maybe this will be a blessing if he dies. No trial. No execution," Stokes said.

"We need to seal up these cases tight all the same. We have CCTV footage of his car at every location. The attack on Fleur Sanders on his property won't be hard to prove, but let's confirm opportunity on the other cases. Don't he and Dr. Marsdon share a receptionist?"

"I'd imagine so," Stokes said. "Want me to check for conflicts in his schedules?"

"We'd better. If by some wild chance he could provide solid alibis for even one murder, it would throw a kink into our case."

Stokes leaned back in his chair, grabbed his notebook, and started to write. "Motives. I can see Jenny Marcus as a crime of passion. The others aren't so clear. Besides, we figured Frankie Campbell for the Detra Ferguson murder because a woman's case file is all that's missing. And why kill Henry Vine and Hermione Jones?"

"We have more work to do. If we can't find the motive for those killings and tie it in with Derren Davide, the DA won't let this one out of the gate."

"Could be that they both were in on all the murders."

"Let's establish a timeline of where each of them was during all four cases," Macy said. He pointed to the whiteboard they used for that purpose. "We find out their appointments, the cell phone records for pinpointing their locations at the time, get a look at their credit card and bank statements for purchases, and anything else that can place either or both of them at the scenes of the crimes. I know we can get warrants for all of that. We have probable cause."

Stokes started to rise, but stopped midway. "What drugs did they find in Derren's bloodwork?"

Macy knew how Stokes thought. How could a drug addict, clumsy enough in his burglary attempt be so adept as to elude them for the murders? "Good question. I have a call in to the police up there. At least we've got him locked up for a crime he can't deny. And he's in no condition to get bail and run."

"You said you were seeing pieces of the day Henry died in your dreams last night."

"Yes," Imogen said. "At first, I thought I had a weird dream about being on a ship, until I remembered the movie I saw that morning. Its' about a woman who loses her husband on a ship, but no one believes her."

Davenport urged her on with a nod.

Session Eight

Imogen sat in the living room, deep into *Dangerous Crossing* playing on TCM when she heard a knock on the front door. Better not to bother Henry. He enjoyed that outdoor work that gave him a break from taking care of her. When she peeked out, she saw Frankie. *What on earth is she doing here?*

"Frankie, hello. Not that I'm not delighted to see you, but I wasn't expecting you."

Frankie, distressed, looked at the driveway before stepping across the threshold. "I wanted to see you. Something's happened, and you're the only close friend I have."

"Come in and sit down. What's happened? Oh, no. It's not Derren again. What has he done to hurt you this time?"

"Don't be like that. You know how careful he has to be. He would go public if he could."

"I don't get it. You're not his patient, for Christ's sake. Who cares if the whole world knows about it? Unless, of course, he's embarrassed of you. I think he's a lying stack of shit. He makes my skin crawl."

"Forget all that for a minute. I have to tell you something important. I need your help. I don't know who else to turn to."

Imogen had reached her limit with this situation that had been going on for over a year. "Okay, what."

"Derren killed that med student you read about in the papers."

"You're not serious?"

"I am. It was a stupid thing to do, but he said it was an accident."

"Tell me this is a joke."

"He asked me to help him. I said I would."

"Like what? Give him an alibi. I guess then he would have to acknowledge you in public."

"Imogen, don't be such a bitch about this. I need you to be on my side."

"I'm not going to help you cover up for that crumb. What's he ever done for me, much less for you that you could expect me to be an accomplice to murder? Honestly, you've lost your mind over this man. That poor girl had a full life ahead besides a brilliant career. How could you justify that?"

"You have to help me. I'm at my wits end. You don't understand all I've done already to protect him. I'm in too far to stop. Please."

"What can I do anyway?"

"I need help to prevent the police from finding out he was the doctor mentoring her."

"Like who?"

"Tate."

Imogen grunted. "Absolutely not. He's our friend. Henry thinks of him like a son."

"I don't mean frame him for murder, but just so the police don't find out about Derren. The cops will look somewhere else, like for a random killer."

"Frankie, I can't help you. I won't call the police, but I'm not doing anything to hurt Tate. You must be crazy to even ask me."

"I see. Well, Imogen. Thanks for being such a good friend. I'll never forgive you for this."

"Neither will I," Imogen said. She watched Frankie stomp out the front door and get into her car. Imogen felt his presence before she knew Henry was behind her.

"We've got to call the police, Imogen. Think of that poor girl and her family. They deserve justice, not a frame up. Think of Tate. How you could live with yourself if

Tate's implicated in a vulgar crime like that? Even if the truth comes out later, the negative publicity could ruin him. People always say, where's there's smoke... You know I'm right."

"I know. Can we wait to call the police until tomorrow? The least I should do is warn her what we're going to do."

"Imogen, you're too gentle and too naïve for your own good. I can't imagine the trouble you'd get into if I weren't around."

When Imogen finished talking, she looked at Dr. Davenport. His lower jaw hung open and he appeared frozen. "Doctor, are you okay?"

"Imogen, we need to call that detective immediately. You need to tell them everything you've remembered here. We have a professional confidence between us, but even I cannot morally justify that confidentiality to cover up a murder."

Imogen did not hesitate. She knew for sure that Frankie still posed a threat to Tate. Maybe her resistance to acknowledging the fall her friend had taken had caused her to suffer the trauma-induced memory loss. "I know you're right. I told Erin about what I saw yesterday. She told me she would call them, and I'm sure she did. Would you call the police for me? Is that all right if I give you permission?"

Dr. Davenport reached for his office phone and looked over to Imogen. "Do you remember the detective's name? Never mind, I'll ask for whoever is in charge of the case." After several transfers, he reached Detective Macy. "This is Dr. Davenport. I don't know if you're aware that Imogen Vine is under my care for evaluation."

"Yes, I saw your name in the official reports."

"Imogen's memories have been surfacing rapidly the last days."

"Yes, that's what I understand. Her attorney called me yesterday with information that's turned out to be very useful. I take it you have something new?"

Dr. Davenport cleared his throat. "Imogen is in my office now. We've finished another session. She remembers the early part of the day of Henry's death."

"Okay, don't keep me in suspense."

"Frankie Campbell went to her home that morning to ask her to help her fabricate a relationship between Jenny Marcus and Dr. Marsdon. She refused, and Ms. Campbell stormed off. Henry Vine overheard the conversation through the open window to the backyard where he had been working. He insisted Imogen call the police, but she wanted to wait until she had time to warn her friend. That's as far as her memories go presently. She wanted you to know."

"This answers a lot of questions. Keep up the good work," Macy said. "Please extend my thanks to Mrs. Vine for her help. She may never know just how much assistance she's giving us."

"I'll do that. I believe you have my cell number if you need anything more. Imogen has given me permission to share her treatment progress."

Dr. Davenport replaced the phone in its cradle and looked to Imogen. "I don't like to speculate, Imogen, but I don't think they still believe your confession."

Imogen felt her own jaw drop.

Tate had not expected to hear from Erin until later in

the day. His medical training told him that his heart could not possibly have skipped a beat, but he smiled at the fun of telling himself it had. "Hey," he said.

"Hey, yourself. I've got the good news, bad news scenario for you."

"Okay, don't keep me hanging. Good news, first."

Erin cleared her throat. "I'm positive that Imogen did not kill Henry."

"Based on what?"

"She met with Davenport again this morning. Now, she remembers that Frankie came to her house to ask for help in framing you for the med student's death. This is the first time we've known Frankie was on the scene. What's more, Henry overheard the conversation through the open window. Frankie must have thought Henry was not home because his car wasn't in the driveway. You see where that leads?"

Tate paused long enough to process this new information.

"You know I really hate it when you do that pause thing. Tell me how you're feeling."

"Mixed. I don't think I understand why she would confess if she hadn't done it."

"Davenport said that she could have witnessed the murder, had a sensory overload, like an overloaded electrical circuit. Then, if someone she trusted kept telling her she did it, she would start to believe it."

"Was this the good news or the bad news?" Tate's earlier excitement fizzled.

"That's the good news. The bad news is we haven't been able to find concrete proof Imogen did *not* do it. Davenport called Macy at Imogen's request to relay the new memories, and then he called me. He said the last memories would be the most difficult to retrieve since he believes that time period holds the traumatic events."

"Have you heard about Derren's accident?"

Erin gasped. "An auto accident?"

"Yes. Running away from the police after he burglarized a surgery center for drugs. I haven't had the chance to tell you about what's happened the last two days. Let's just say he's not the man I thought he was."

"You were beginning to think he was a slimy double-dealer."

"Right. It's turned out he's a lot worse."

"Seriously? Tell me about it tonight?"

"Absolutely," Tate said.

"Hold on. Macy's calling," Erin said.

Tate chided himself for feeling abandoned. He did the same thing many times when he saw a call from the hospital, and expected understanding. He considered disconnecting and calling her later when she returned to his call.

"You'll never guess what he wanted, so I won't ask you to try. He wants Imogen to act as bait to get Frankie to admit her involvement in the murders."

"Murders? What other murders?"

"I'm sorry, love. A lot has happened in the last twenty-four hours on my end, too. Macy and his partner found links to four murders, starting with Jenny Marcus, and then Delia Ferguson, Henry, and Hermione. Nothing solid yet, but Frankie's attempt to implicate you at the police station brought the focus on her. They started thinking on those lines before any help from Imogen."

"When is this set up happening? They're not going to let you be there, I hope."

"This evening. I insisted I be allowed to be there, but I have to stay back Frankie's been trying to get in to see Imogen since she's been in custody. Macy believes she wants to make sure Imogen never remembers. He's counting on her to make some kind of acknowledgment that will tie her to Henry's murder. Davenport discussed it with Imogen before he called me."

"So Imogen agreed to this? It sounds dangerous. If Frankie *is* a killer, wouldn't her solution be to kill Imogen?"

"Imogen's anxious to find the truth. Yes, she knows there's an element of danger, but she believes she can pull it off. The police will have a recording device in the visitor's room and be in the next room," Erin said. "If it works out, they'll arrest Frankie. There's still the question of who did the actual killings, but if they can get her to implicate herself, Macy believes the rest of the truth will follow."

"That's a brave thing Imogen's doing," Tate said.

"Yes, but she also has a lot to lose. It's a risk worth taking." Erin said. "Now, what did Derren do?"

"I don't know which is worse, the corpse harvesting or stealing drugs from our practice."

"You're kidding. Are you sure? He doesn't have the look of someone on drugs. And not even in my wildest dreams would I imagine him being so creepy as to use recycled parts on a patient."

"On the first account, I can't say he uses drugs, but he steals them. On the second, I found his handiwork inside a patient."

"Holy cow. I've read about those other cases in New York and Texas. If the patients have a choice, that's one thing, but to learn you're carrying around something stolen from a dead person is plain mortifying. Then to tack murder on top of that, he'll be lucky if he sees daylight without bars the rest of his life."

Tate examined his emotions. His rage resurfaced, but

he had to be honest with himself. Was he angry with Derren for his actions, or was he angrier that he had not been able to spot the problems before he could prevent them?

"Are you there?" Erin said.

"Yes, I had to take a minute. I'm keeping my temper under control, but it's not easy." This time, Erin went silent. He went on. "Thanks for not saying you told me so."

"I would *never*," Erin said.

"Right," Tate said. "How are you taking this new information about Hermione?"

"If we've found the who, I'd still like to know the why."

"Has to be a case of mistaken identity. If it turns out to be Derren or Frankie, that could only mean a connection with Imogen. You're her attorney. You know me. You have a reputation for getting to the truth, and that might have scared them."

"How am I supposed to live with knowledge that she's dead because of me? Her loss leaves a hole that can never be filled again."

"I'm sorry," Tate said.

"No, I'm sorry. I forgot you lost a close friend, too."

"What time is this thing happening with Imogen?"

"Macy said Davenport will notify Frankie that Imogen can have visitors. He expects she'll come right away, but he didn't have a timeline."

"Now that Derren is incapacitated in the hospital, I'm going to do more digging into his files at the office to find out how deep this goes. Call when you have news."

Monica and Devon sat next to Fleur's hospital bed.

She had not woken up yet, but the doctors said that head injuries are like that. They expected her to wake up, but they had no way to tell about the extent of the damage to her brain until then. Monica looked at Devon and wondered if they were thinking the same thing. If only Devon had not had that doctor's appointment, one of them would have been with Fleur, or at least talked her out of it. If only Fleur had texted one of them about where Frankie went.

"It's easier in retrospect," Devon said.

Monica jumped. "What?"

"That's what you're thinking, isn't it? All the ways this could have ended better. You play the what-if game for everything, and I can see it in your face."

"You're right. I need to stop that, but I'm broken-hearted that this happened to her."

They looked at Fleur at the same time. She looked like a soiled angel from her prone position, gravity pulling back any wrinkles she had, her pouty lips partly opened as if she were preparing to speak. She had been fortunate the head wounds had been from the side with only one severe laceration to her forehead. She had a broken nose from the attack or from hitting her face when she landed face down onto the black top where the police found her. Dr. Tate stitched up her cuts and reset her nose once the other surgeons took care of the more serious injuries to the rest of her body.

"Fleur would be pleased to know she's still attractive after what she's had been through," Devon said. They both smiled.

"I want to kill Frankie," Monica said. "This is all her fault."

"Do we know that for a fact?"

Monica rolled her eyes. "It's obvious. Fleur followed

her, Frankie saw her, and did this. I know it."

"You feel it, but you don't know it yet."

"Devon, you're getting on my nerves, and that makes me feel guilty. Knock it off."

Devon let out a victorious laugh and winked at Monica.

"Can't you guys see I'm trying to sleep here?" Fleur's voice, weak and groggy, startled them.

"Fleur, you're awake! Thank God," Monica said. Devon pressed the button for the nurse—neither wanted to move away. "How do you feel?"

"I feel terrible. What happened? Is this a hospital? Oh my God." The conscious Fleur started to touch her face and then ran her hands down her body in a panic.

"Fleur, stop moving like that. The nurse will be here in a minute. You took a terrible beating, but you're going to be fine. You're going to take time to heal." Monica watched tears pool in Fleur's eyes.

"What about my face?"

Monica and Devon let out laughs. "Dr. Tate took care of you. He'll give you the gory details, but he said you wouldn't have a scar."

"I guess you wouldn't laugh if it were more serious, right?" Fleur relaxed into her pillows about the time the nurse entered.

"You girls have to leave now. I need to take her vitals. I'll call the doctor to tell him the patient is awake, and he'll be in to check on her. Why not go to the cafeteria and have a bite? Then you can come back."

Monica turned back to Fleur. "We'll be back in a half hour. Don't get into any trouble while we're gone."

"Oh, don't make me laugh. It hurts."

Monica took Devon's arm and led her to the hallway.

"We need to call Detective Macy right away."

CHAPTER TWENTY TWO

Macy received a call from the hospital that Fleur Sanders had woken up. Under normal circumstances, he would have rushed right over, but this meeting between Imogen and Frankie took precedence. They could get a confession on tape that could solve four murders. Fleur's statements would only confirm his, hers, or both motivations.

The technician set the recording device and small camera in the visitor's room. Macy, Stokes, Erin and two officers sat in the next room. He locked the door and shut off the lights. Fortunately, the window gave them light until dusk. They sat in silence. Macy hated waiting. Sitting in one spot through long hours of surveillance made him stiff. He hoped this went quickly.

Frankie dropped everything to leave for the hospital when Dr. Davenport called to tell her that Imogen could see her. She kept her pace light and smooth from the parking lot to the nurse's station. A genial woman who looked about her age greeted her.

"I'm Frankie Campbell. I'm here to see Imogen Vine."

"Yes, Ms. Campbell, Imogen is waiting for you in the visitor's lounge down this hallway and to the left. You'll see the sign."

Frankie's heels on the shiny tiles echoed so loudly in

this quiet corridor, she thought of taking off her shoes. She saw the sign above a door that she had arrived at her destination. She paused, and then opened the door.

Imogen stood by the window. When she turned around, Frankie gaped at the hollow look in her face—strained and exhausted. She had not looked this bad when she had cancer. Frankie's conscience pinged her while she stood there, but by the time she reached Imogen, the alien sensation had left her.

"Imogen, I'm so happy I've finally been allowed to see you. How are you holding up?"

After a deep breath, Imogen said, "I'm okay. I'm getting better every day, and I have a great doctor helping me with my memory loss."

Frankie noted the tone in that pointed remark. "Oh, that's good."

"Yes, it is good. I had lost memories going back all year. But in every meeting with him, Dr. Davenport draws out more."

"How far have you gotten?"

"Up to the day of Henry's death." Frankie could not meet Imogen's eye for long. Imogen's intense stare forced her to turn away. She had not anticipated that Imogen would be this strong, or could this be anger? She calculated her next move.

"What do you remember?"

"I remember you visited me that day. I remember you wanted me to help you frame Tate for the med student's murder." Imogen's eyes had turned red.

"I see. Anything else?"

"I remember enough to know I didn't kill my husband. I think you killed Henry."

Frankie reared back from the caustic tone in Imogen's voice, and the accusation.

"Just tell me why. You knew how much he meant to me. What could be so important that you would rob me of that?"

"Imogen, you're wrong. You killed Henry."

"No I didn't. No matter how many arguments we had, I would never have done that to myself or to our children."

Frankie studied Imogen's face for clues. What did she remember, and what could she really prove? Who would believe her if she knew the whole truth?

"You know why. He wanted you to call the police. I couldn't have that."

"Why, because the world would learn that your precious Derren murdered that poor girl at the airport?"

"No, because the world would learn that I killed her."

Imogen gasped. "Oh…my…God!"

"That's what Henry heard when I came back later."

"How could you do that? To anyone?"

"It started out that I only meant to follow him to find out if he were seeing someone. When I saw them argue and he attacked her, I was glad. I thought he had killed her until I got to her car and saw her rubbing her throat. She didn't know me, so she rolled down the window to ask what I wanted. I reached in and finished the job."

Frankie looked out the window to calm down. "I found it amusing that he wanted me to help him cover his murder. At first, I felt awful about killing the stupid little fool, and made the mistake of telling my therapist. I had told her too much, so I had to kill her, too."

"Frankie, what's happened to you? I can't believe you're so casual about what you've done." Imogen started to back away from her. "Don't tell me you killed Erin's friend, too?"

"That was a mistake. How did I know she'd have an

out of town visitor?"

"Frankie, I think you've gone insane. Just tell me why—what's it all about?"

"Imogen, you'll never understand how it feels to be so bulletproof no man can ever get through. For the first time in years, an attractive man found me appealing."

"But he used you. He was ashamed to acknowledge you in public. What kind of love is that?"

"It's what I could get, so I took it. Now, that's all over. Without him, I have little to lose."

"But you have the restaurant. You have money. You could do anything you want."

"Money," Frankie laughed. "That just builds a doorway that lets the devil in."

"I feel sorry for you, Frankie. I had no idea you were so pathetic."

"I don't need your pity. All I need is for you to stop remembering. Without you blabbing everything to the cops, they won't have enough evidence to prove I did anything."

"Who's going to stop me? You?"

Frankie reached into her satchel and pulled out a syringe. She pulled the protective plastic tip from the needle and started toward Imogen. "What's in here will make you seem like an idiot who lost her memory again. Who'll believe anything you have to say after that."

"What's that?" Imogen started backing up to get to the door.

"It's called Ketamine. I stole some from a vet's office. They use it to sedate pets."

"Frankie, no. Please don't do this."

"I'm only interested in surviving, and you're blocking my path." Frankie moved faster toward her. Imogen grabbed a metal chair and whacked Frankie on the right side with all her strength. Frankie staggered, lost her balance, and started to drop to the floor. Her hands flailed as she tried to block her fall with her hands. She still clutched the syringe. The erratic movements of her hands to find something to break her fall rammed the needle into her hip when her head hit the floor.

"Damn," Frankie said before she lost consciousness.

Imogen reeled backed in relief. She placed her hand over her chest to check her racing heart. Macy and Stokes crashed through the door followed by the rest of his team. Erin rushed to her and took her in her arms.

"What took you so long?" Imogen said. "I've never been so scared in my life."

"We didn't count on her bracing the door shut. She must've wanted to be sure no one interrupted her giving that injection."

The two officers picked Frankie up from the floor, still conscious but obviously intoxicated. The technician rushed out to get help, and returned with two men carrying a stretcher.

"One of these officers will follow you and stand guard until she's coherent enough to be arrested and sent downtown," Stokes said. He nodded to the male nurses to signal them to go, and watched them carried Frankie through the narrow doorway.

"Did you hear everything?" Imogen still clung to Erin.

"We sure did. Everything is on video and recorder."

"I can't believe I didn't break down."

"You did better than I would have," Erin said.

"You were great," Stokes said. "I almost believed you remembered everything."

"What's going to happen to me now?"

"You're free as far as we're concerned," Macy said. "But you should meet with Dr. Davenport again. You've been through a lot this evening."

"He's right, Imogen," Erin said. "Take advantage of the help while you can. After hearing Frankie talk of murder in that casual way, I might need help."

"You're right. It must have been as harsh to hear about your friend as it was for me to hear about my Henry."

Erin did not answer, but held on to Imogen in a tighter embrace.

Now that she had the confrontation behind her, Imogen broke down crying.

"We're sorry for your losses. It can't have been easy being in here, unable to be with friends and family. At least now the worst is over."

"I appreciate you saying that. I need to go to my room and fall apart. I haven't come to terms with what just happened yet."

CHAPTER TWENTY THREE

Fleur winced when Macy and Stokes entered her room. Her injuries had made it difficult, if not impossible, to shift her body without pain. She wondered what lame pain meds pumped through her IV, because their effects diminished every hour. Or so it seemed to her. Every twinge, every tender spot made her determined to strangle Frankie within seconds from death, then bring her back just to beat her to a pulp. Her agitation fueled her awareness of pain, an effect the nurse warned her against due to increasing her heart rate and lessening the delivery of the medication. *The nurse might have something there.*

"We're glad to hear you're going to be okay," Macy said.

"Me, too. I heard they're booting me out of here soon. I'll be glad to be home. I've got nothing to do here but think of revenge. From the moment I came around, it's the only thing that seems to matter."

Stokes gave out a snort. "You'll have to get in line. She's in custody. Four counts of murder. We need your statement to confirm the assault, and then we'll add that charge. Unless she gets out of this by an act of God, she's spending the rest of her life in prison, if she's lucky *not* to get the death penalty."

"Four murders? I can't take that in. That doesn't make sense. She had everything going for her. She could be bitchy at times, but tolerable. Why?"

"Apparently for love," Macy said.

"Derren?" Fleur said. "She never did have any sense when it came to men. I'm glad she's in jail. The picture of her out there, free to have another try to kill me had me anxious. What a relief."

"Nurse Ratched out there told us to be brief, so we better get on with this. If you can give us your account of what happened, we can get out of here, and let you rest." Stokes winked at Fleur, and drew her smile.

Macy cleared his throat and pulled out his notepad. "Ready when you are, Miss."

Fleur rested her eyes on Stokes longer than she intended and then turned to Macy. "I followed her to confirm my suspicion that she had someone in her life that she kept hidden from us."

"What made you suspect that?" Macy said.

"Her bizarre behavior talking against Dr. Tate, for one thing. She's always an opinionated bitch, but implying he killed Jenny Marcus went way past the mark. I knew someone else had to be at the bottom of this, so I camped outside her restaurant that night to follow her and see if she met up with someone."

"She drove directly to Durango Hills?" Macy said.

"Right. I couldn't believe it when I realized she drove to Dr. Davide's house."

"You took quite a risk walking up to the property like that," Stokes said.

Fleur ignored his remark. "I thought I took precautions. I couldn't just park out in the open, so I found a place to conceal my car behind a tree a few houses down the road. I walked back and went around to the side yard. I saw a window with light, so I tiptoed toward it and looked in. I can tell you I lost any remaining respect I had for Dr. Davide when I saw him kissing Miss Iron Britches."

"Which window?" Macy said.

"On the south side, the one that looks into the dining room through to the living room."

"Okay, go on."

"I guess I got excited and forgot to be careful. I took out my phone to take pictures. They must've heard me or saw the light on the phone. The next thing I knew they ran out of the front door and cornered me." Fleur's face contorted.

"I didn't have time to say anything before Frankie produced a cricket bat out of nowhere and whacked me on my back. I staggered but didn't fall. She hit me again. This time, I fell down on my knees. That's when she kept hitting me with that damn thing. When she whacked me on the side of my head, I lost control and dropped to the ground."

"Take it easy," Stokes said. "Reliving memories can be as real as when you experienced them."

Fleur welcomed the break. She looked over to Stokes with a grateful smile. She took a deep breath that hurt her bruised body more than calmed her and then continued.

"I pretended to be unconscious so she she'd stop the attack. I heard Derren say, what were you thinking? I can't have her found here. Get rid of her. I don't care how. Just do it."

"Then he went into the house and left her outside with me. I could have taken her then, but I didn't feel I could take another blow if I were wrong. I let her drag me into the garage. She left me for a few minutes. Another opportunity to try to get away, but I didn't know how far I'd get in my condition. He returned with her, and they lifted me into the back seat of her car."

Stokes interrupted her. "Didn't they wonder about your car?"

"Not that I heard," she said.

"Okay," Stokes said. "Go on."

"There I was in the backseat, positive they would notice me breathing. All I could think to do was to stay still. They had a few heated words before he went back inside. She got in the car, and drove a long time before she stopped. She opened the car door and pulled me out of the car feet first. I remember the pain of my head hitting the ground. I guess I'm lucky she didn't run over me when she drove off. Even spread out on that blacktop in the middle of the night, I finally felt out of danger. I sort of let go. Today is the first memory since then."

Macy had been writing, but looked up when she stopped talking. "We've kept you long enough. I'm sorry we had to ask you to go through it all."

"It's worth it if it keeps her in jail."

"Don't worry. We won't let anything happen to you," Stokes said. His deep voice came out sultry and intimate.

Fleur tingled with a flirtatious excitement and smiled wide in spite of her facial injuries. She wiggled a couple of fingers at them when they left the room. If she could be interested in a man in her present condition, she knew she would live.

Tate called to get the status of Derren's condition from the trauma doctor in charge of his case.

"He didn't do himself any favors by driving like a maniac straight into the biggest ass Saguaro in Arizona." The doctor on the other end of the line chuckled. "He wasn't wearing a seatbelt either. His head crashed into the windshield when the vehicle hit the cactus, causing traumatic head injury. We know from the X-rays that he has extensive bleeding and swelling inside the brain. He's been in surgery to take care of the brain bleed."

Tate listened to the details in the detached manner he had when he consulted with the ER doctors on other patients. His lack of emotional attachment surprised him.

"He also has fractured ribs and punctured lungs. No other injuries in that area. A femoral fracture, as well as fractures in both ankles and knees from when the knee well collapsed around his lower extremities. He'll need reconstruction for his jaw and dental injuries, and for the extensive lacerations from the windshield. You'll be relieved to hear we didn't find drugs in his system."

"Yeah," Tate said. "Relieved is the word."

"What about next of kin? We haven't found an emergency contact."

Somehow, talk of family, implying somewhere in the world someone had concern for Derren's wellbeing made him less of a villain. "He has a mother overseas. I can find her contact information on his computer at the office."

"I'd appreciate that. Are you planning to come over here?"

"No, but the police probably will. I appreciate the update"

The other end of the line went quiet for several moments. "I assumed him being your partner…"

"Thanks," Tate said. He disconnected and sat back. He grudgingly admitted he was glad Derren survived, but his unconscious condition left too many questions unanswered.

CHAPTER TWENTY FOUR

Imogen looked down at her lap, her hands clasped, her knees touching to keep them from shaking. The idea of going back into the real world seemed a menacing proposition. Sure, she looked forward to seeing her friends, but going back to her life without Henry did not seem worth living, if she were honest with herself. The tears were coming back. Vicious spasms assaulted her body whenever she allowed her mind to see the last look of her home before they led her out to the police car. Worse than that, she kept seeing the image of the stretcher carrying Henry's dead body when it passed her in the living room. Until that moment, she had made herself believe Henry was still alive. At least, Dr. Davenport explained it that way yesterday after the big scene.

A nurse came in, this one younger and perkier than the others. Imogen thought how wonderful it had been to be that age with her life spread out in front of her. The intoxication of life. To be happy, optimistic, and determined to live life well. She returned the smile and took a seat in the wheelchair. The movement created a slight breeze that caught the ends of her hair. She touched the side of her head, cringed at the stiff ends, and chided herself for not thinking of a hat sooner.

The elevator doors opened and the nurse pushed the chair forward. The motions around her confused her.

Imogen tried to focus in on one thing, but so many people standing, rushing, or strolling down different corridors or between the modern seating around the information desk made her head swim. She gripped the armrests for stability from the dizzying effect of sudden activity after her isolation. Then she heard familiar voices.

She had not noticed them sitting on one of the sofas when she glanced in that direction the first time. Monica wore a nose splint. Fleur barely able to walk upright held onto Devon who looked tired like an overworked caregiver.

"Where's your luggage?" Devon looked serious, but Imogen giggled.

"Don't be a stereotype, Devon," Fleur said. "This hasn't been a stay at a five-star hotel."

Monica took Imogen's hand and gave her a wide smile. "How are you, sweetie? I've missed you."

"Looks like I'm better off than the two of you. Devon, what happened to these characters?"

Devon opened her mouth, but Monica held up her hand.

"I got this," Monica said, pointing to her nose splint, "when Troy flipped me over and right off the side of the bed last night."

"You didn't tell us that when we asked earlier." Fleur gave Monica a suspicious glare.

"It's embarrassing, and I needed time to figure out how to spin it."

Devon had the look of sheer terror on her face, her eyes wide and mouth hanging open.

"Devon, close your jaw," Monica said.

"Does this kind of thing happen to you a lot?"

Monica gave Devon a severe look. "It was an accident. See, this is why I'm not telling anyone else."

"What a scene that must've been," Fleur said. "I won't be able to look at Troy again without that visual."

Imogen laughed, enjoying the exchange among them. So natural, so much in character that for a few minutes she forgot her anxiety, but then they went quiet.

"Come on, ladies," Monica said. "Let's get you out of this invalid chair and blow this joint."

When they reached the exit, Imogen stood up. The idea of going outside panicked her. She thought of sitting down until she turned to see the back of the attendant pushing it out of her reach.

"You're good," Fleur said.

"I don't know if anything will ever be good for me again." For Imogen, images of her past swirled in front of her, blinding her in a blanket of white. Then the future loomed over her head, menacing and suffocating like she would smother inside its darkness. "I'm sorry for losing it just then. It all rushed over me like I'd been hit in the stomach."

"You've nothing to be sorry about," Fleur said. "We understand. Honestly."

"Right, into the car," Monica said. "I'm taking you home with me for a few days. Lord knows I've got no work on right now, so I've plenty of time to hang out with you."

"I'm not resisting. I'll never be able to go inside my own house again."

"Let's go to the Court for a long lunch," Fleur said. "Then Monica can tell us all about what exactly one has to be doing to get thrown out of bed during sex."

Monica watched the three other women laughing, drinking wine like water, and tossing artery-clogging double Machaca nachos like target practice past their continuously moving lips. The sight pleased her, but more as a sign of their resilience than the celebration to the end of an ordeal that none of them could wipe from their memories. The experience imprinted them in different ways, but Monica knew the one constant had to be the loss of their innocence toward violence. She shuddered and blinked hard.

"So Monica, we're waiting for details," Fleur said.

"You know she won't let it go until you do," Imogen said.

Devon rolled her eyes. "I don't know if I want to hear this."

"You're too sheltered, Devon," Fleur said. "This will be a good way to get some pointers."

"Yes, Devon," Monica said. "You've got to stop treating men like dogs. You know, like the Dog Whisperer says, "No talk, no touch, no eye contact.""

"I don't do that."

"Of course you do, but that's okay. One of us should be sweet and innocent in this group."

Monica smiled back at their amused faces, and then their eyes focused on something behind her. She swung around to see Tate standing there, grinning.

"I think they're teasing you, Monica." Tate said. "Did you forget you invited me? You look surprised."

"Sorry, I did forget," Monica said. Reddening at the memory when she explained the accident to nurses and others in the ER last night before Tate arrived. "Have my seat. I'll get the waiter to bring another over."

She got up and left the table before anyone could protest. She followed the waiter back with the extra chair, she sat next to Tate, hoping the conversation had moved on since she left.

"Monica, it's not so bad," Tate said.

"But everyone who spoke to me acted as if they didn't believe me. When they saw Troy, they treated him like a criminal. How humiliating. I felt like a fool."

"What you don't see is how many battered women come in for treatment after a beating, sometimes with the abusive man standing next to her. She makes up excuses for what's happened, and refuses to notify the police. The hospital staff goes out of their way to get the women to admit what happened, but only to protect them. You'd be surprised how many women lie and end up there again."

"Monica, chill," Fleur said. "We're just having fun with you. Forget about it."

An abrupt silence emerged between them. Monica knew he needed to make peace with Imogen, and possibly Imogen needed the same.

"Tate, I'm sorry for the problems I caused you." Imogen spoke like a broken woman. "I know I had a break with reality, but I can't help but think that if I'd called the police when Frankie first told me what she was up to, Henry would still be alive, so would Erin's friend, and I wouldn't have lost my sanity. I'll carry that regret with me the rest of my life."

At first, Monica thought he was not going to say anything. He hesitated as he did so often in the office when asked a serious medical question. She remembered how crazy that made her, waiting for him to speak, wanting to drag out the words or say them for him. This time, she welcomed the hesitation, afraid of what he would say. She had never known him to evade a direct question, and sometimes his honesty could sting.

"Imogen," he said. "I don't blame you. Of course, when I thought you killed Henry, I wanted you punished. But as the case was building against me, your loyalty to me caused you to fight through your breakdown to warn me about Frankie and Derren's plot. If you had not been observant, you might have missed seeing Frankie and Derren together which started to tie the truth together."

Monica felt the onset of a crying jag. She looked at Imogen. When she saw her crying, she avoided looking at the others. Crying is contagious. Wine did not mix with emotion.

Fleur leaned in. "How's Erin?"

Tate shifted. For the first time, Monica saw discomfort in his mannerisms. Understandable. Hermione turned out to be collateral damage. If Erin had not represented Imogen, her best friend would be alive now. Monica kept her opinions from Tate and her friends, because she was not certain she could forgive easily if she were in Erin's position.

"She's pleased things worked out for you, of course," he said. "She's accompanying Hermione back to their hometown for burial."

Monica glanced at Imogen, who had stopped smiling. Yes, she thought, Imogen felt the same way. That Erin had her to blame for this. Monica had no doubt the others had the same idea.

"This is my fault," Imogen said. "There can't be a truly happy ending when you can't undo an injustice."

Tate looked like he had gone into a meditative state, but he looked over to Imogen. "Blaming yourself won't bring anyone back. Anyway, if anyone should take the blame, it's Frankie and Derren. And I have to take some of the blame for not keeping a closer eye on what my partner was doing. The truth is all of us were fooled."

"What's happening to Derren now?" Fleur said. "Hasn't he been arrested yet?"

"You can't arrest an unconscious person," Monica

said.

"When can the cops get on with it?"

"Hard to say," Tate said. "He sustained massive injuries, not to mention the head trauma. They can't assess the effect that had on the brain until he's conscious. No one can say definitively at this point."

"Is he allowed visitors?" Fleur said.

The others looked at her with surprise.

"Why? You can't think of visiting him?" Devon said.

"I'd like the opportunity to flip off the switch to his life support. My way of thanking him for the beating I took." Fleur's face tightened, her eyes dilated. Monica was sure she was fantasizing again, but not in a good way.

"I'll assume you're joking," Tate said.

"Sure, I am," Fleur said. "but I'd want a crack at the cow first."

Monica looked at Tate. "She's not really serious. It makes her feel better. Her way of coping."

Tate looked skeptical, but did not respond. "Listen, I can't stay. I'm taking Erin to the airport this afternoon." He looked down at his watch. "I need to leave now."

He stood up to go. He hugged each of them until he reached Imogen. He hesitated at first, and then he watched her rise up to wrap her arms around his neck and bury her face in the folds of his shirt.

"I'm so sorry," she said.

"It's okay, Imogen. Really." He pulled away and left them watching his moving figure exit the patio into the bar.

"I need some giggle juice," Fleur said and waved for the waiter.

"It occurs to me that Tate has lost more than anyone else in the mess." Devon, the one who could not compete with the forceful nature of the others, spoke in an authoritarian tone that caught the group's attention. "He lost a close friend, Henry." She nodded to Imogen. "Then he lost a partner, even if they weren't close. There might be fallout for his practice from the publicity, even if he did nothing wrong. Finally, there's, Hermione. He might lose Erin over this."

CHAPTER TWENTY FIVE

Tate pulled up in front of Erin's condo building to park when he saw her leaning on the edge of a flowerbed, her luggage standing next to her. Before she noticed him, he saw a frailty he had not recognized before. The momentary glimpse of her inner pain pulled at him. She was suffering, but this time he could not find the right words or actions to make her feel better. When she saw him watching, she shifted her expression like pulling on an imaginary mask to cover her vulnerability.

He took her bags, put them in the trunk, and then opened her door. She slid in effortlessly one leg at a time, and when he saw the flash of inner thigh exposed when the light silk material of her shorts fluttered from a sudden breeze, he forgot everything except the memory of running his hands across her naked skin. She settled, looking up at him with questioning eyes that reminded him of intimate times when she looked up at him, her eyes boring into him, her mouth partly open, anticipating him.

"What's wrong?"

"Nothing," he said. He knew his face had that sudden flush. He had to stay focused. This was not the time. He closed her door, walked around to make sure he closed the trunk, and started the short drive to the airport.

"I know what you're thinking," she said. "That I'm breaking down finally."

"No, that's not what I was thinking." A wave of guilt rushed over him when he could not take his mind or his eyes from her inner thighs.

"I've seen this happen to clients after they've been exonerated. First, they have the ecstatic high, but the physical stress they endured throughout the court proceedings finally takes over. Some have even come down with serious illnesses. The difference is I recognize what's happening. I'm mourning my loss as best as I can. Having the service and the burial ceremony will help me."

"Are you sure you don't want me to come with you?"

"I'm sure. Anyway, you can't be away from your practice right now. I'll be fine. It's my last road trip with Hermione."

Tate heard the crack in her voice, but pretended he did not notice. "When will you be back?"

"Soon. No longer than a week. I have my own clients to take care of."

He ran out of gentle small talk, and he guessed she did too. Neither of them spoke the rest of the way. He kept making sideward glances at her lap, and had a difficult time thinking of anything else. He pacified himself that this had to be his way of deflecting grief.

When they reached the airport, he parked and walked inside with her. While she checked her bags, he watched her deal with the attendant. She asserted her independence and strength of will during a dispute she had with the other woman. When she turned back, she had the vitality he knew her for. Maybe going on her own was the best thing. Relying on him would weaken her, a realization that gave him a pang of sadness for the limits of their relationship.

"Well, this is it for now," she said. "It's too bad this isn't the old days when you could walk me to the gate and sit with me until boarding."

"Who even remembers that anymore?" He touched her chin, and she moved her face to meet his. He kissed her forehead, then her nose, and then brushed his lips against hers. She pulled away to look him in the eye. He thought she had become conscious of their public display of intimacy until she kissed him back.

"I don't blame you," she said. "You know that, right?"

"I can't see how you can't blame me. It's because of me you were involved."

"That's true, but look at it this way. If I didn't know you, I might still have taken her case. The same thing could've happened."

"That's a big *if.*"

"I'm still angry and hurt on many levels, but maybe this was Hermione's time."

"You can't believe that," he said.

"I have to."

He knew what she meant. The loss had to make sense so she could deal with it. That was not his style, but who could say she was wrong.

She gave him another kiss, this time more forceful, and winked as she started to walk away. "I'll be back before you have time to miss me." He watched her make her way to the security line before turning back to his car. He knew she was wrong because he missed her already.

EPILOGUE

Erin had been right. Except for their time in the airport, he had little time since then to miss her or to meditate on the events of the past few weeks. Being on call this week, he had not had one free evening. During the weekdays, he saw patients in his office, met with his accountants and lawyers about the state of the practice and his legal obligations while extricating himself from his partnership with Derren. When he thought about his week, he realized he could not remember the last time he ate, so he headed toward the cafeteria.

The hospital sounds at five in the morning, both muted and intermittent, soothed him. He walked along the corridor, his eyes burning from the long procedure he finished a half hour before. The tiredness would kick in if he let it, so he kept his mind on tasks for tomorrow. No, today, this morning, a few hours from now. Another long day ahead.

"Good morning, doctor." He turned to see Judy, one of the cooks, loading up for the breakfast rush, exchanging out the sandwiches for breakfast rolls and bagels. "You've been here all night?"

"Yeah. And I haven't eaten."

"You need a wholesome bowl of oatmeal? That'll stick to your ribs."

"That sounds good."

"I know how you like strawberries. I'll stir some in. How about an apple to take with you?"

"You're too good to me, Judy."

"Not hard to do. We all think a lot of you around here."

Some days, simple shows of appreciation inspired him to keep moving. He sat at a table in the corner where he found the morning newspaper and began to skim through the headlines.

"Dr. Magnus Onderdonk. Please call admitting."

Tate laughed out loud. *Where did he get a name like that?* Magnus, who some of the nurses called Magnum for his dark Germanic good looks, had all the charm of a rectal thermometer, but had the mistaken idea that he was irresistible to women. It was unfortunate that the female staff had not gotten that memo. Tate tried to avoid the man who liked to give gruesome details of his sexual conquests during surgery, or anywhere he had a captive audience. His one sensitive spot, the only thing, according to him that slowed his professional progress, was his last name. The last time they got trapped in a slow elevator, he told Tate he was working on changing his name. He just had to find the right name to suit him.

"Dr. Magnus Onders, you're needed in Emergency Room One."

"We don't have two doctors with that name. What's he up to?" Tate looked up at the recessed speaker delivering the monotone message. Two more messages followed closely. One with the name, Dr. Mark Onders, and then Dr. Merit Odon. Tate rolled his eyes. He did not like either of those. He knew this had to be him practicing the sound of his name.

Magnus must have decided on a whole new approach, because the next page was for Mark Malik, then another for Martin Olson. Tate wondered what the operator thought of all this, or if he had lured her into these hospital hijinks as a coconspirator. Finally, the serial pages stopped. Tate finished his oatmeal, and the paper, and stuffed the apple in his jacket pocket. If he hurried, he could get home, have a shower and a quick doze before his first office appointment.

Tate nodded to Judy, who was busy serving now, and walked toward the front door to the garage. With rest in his sights, he reached into his pockets and had just touched the familiar metal of his keychain when someone called out his name. The urgency in the shrill voice startled him.

"Doctor Marsdon, please come. There's been a horrible *incident*." He recognized the nurse, another one of Onderdonk's conquests. She looked pale and frightened, suddenly aware of the staring eyes from passersby. She lowered her voice. "Please, something horrible has happened."

In an uncharacteristic gesture, she grabbed his arm to instigate action.

"What's happened?"

"Not here. I don't want to panic the patients."

He let her lead him down the corridor to a vacant room. He felt irritable. What did the fool do this time? He knew this had to be something to do with Onderdonk. He pushed the door open and motioned for her to lead. She looked up at him to protest, but started in when she saw his disapproving look.

"I was supposed to meet Magnus here for...Well, anyway, I got delayed about ten minutes. When I walked in, the room was dark and I thought he got ticked and left. I started to leave when I saw the edge of his coat sticking out." She pointed at the floor beyond the second bed. He could see how she almost missed him.

He walked over and looked down. Magnus Onderdonk would not have to worry about his name ever again.

ACKNOWLEDGEMENTS

First, I must thank Pablo Andres Prichard, MD, Director of Plastic and Reconstructive Surgery at John C Lincoln Hospital, and senior partner at Advanced Aesthetics Associates in Phoenix and Scottsdale, Arizona, for providing technical advice and occasional anecdotes for the storyline that made this book better than its original inception.

My appreciation to Pamela Holland, MD, of VA Medical Center Emergency Department in Lexington, Kentucky, for having the first read and finding the error that saved me from overdosing Tate's patient.

I also want to thank Margaret Morse for contributing her legal expertise.

Finally, thanks to Elizabeth, Diane, Fran, Phyllis, and Joan, the most important contributors, who shared their breast cancer experiences with me over the years, and inspired me to find a way to share their story.

Thanks for reading my book. If you enjoyed it, please take a moment to leave me a review at your favorite online-retailer.

Connect with me on Social Sites

Twitter: https://twitter.com/feywritinggirl
Facebook:
https://www.facebook.com/cathyannrogers
LinkedIn: www.linkedin.com/in/cathyannrogers
Website: http://www.cathyannrogers.com

Discover other titles by Cathy Ann Rogers

Deliberate Fools
Here Lies Buried
Heavy Mascara A Short Story Collection
Cat Pistol Hoodlum, A Short Story

ABOUT THE AUTHOR

CATHY ANN ROGERS has a penchant for creating literary characters who imitate reality through their skewed sense of justice as well as their bittersweet victories.

Cathy attributes the shaping of her writer's prowess to her solitary upbringing as an only child. Armed with a library card from her neighborhood branch in Cincinnati, she spent her childhood absorbed in suspenseful scenes depicted within the fiction of Christie and Conan-Doyle. Simultaneously, she built a mental library of potential plots while eavesdropping on the conversations of adults who discussed everything from Hollywood to History. The result of these blended influences is her fascination with plot twists and multi-generational storytelling in novels.

Following the dictates of her left-brain, Cathy pursued a degree and graduate certificate in accounting, establishing a tax and bookkeeping service for entrepreneurs.

Cathy weaves her tales from her Arizona desert townhome in the company of her Bichon Frises, Whitney and Sophie. She is currently working on the next installment of the Pilar Sagasta series *Here Lies Hidden*.

Excerpt from,

Here Lies Hidden
A Pilar Sagasta Mystery

Prologue

St Petersburg, Russia 1914 Royal Palace

Madame Natalia Rosenlof leaned into her companion's neck space, and whispered, "That woman has more than one murder coming to her." The sultry voice spit out that remark as the smoke oozed from her nose and mouth, the breathy words an audible irony to Madame Natalia's visual refinement. Sonya held no judgment against her friend and benefactor, knowing the audacious nature of, Princess Anastasia, the woman in question now holding court with various young military admirers.

From across the room, the two women watched and listened to endless flirtatious witticisms between the princess and the young men who vied for her attentions.

This is what one must do, Madame Natalia had told Sonya. A woman must be cordial in society; deny the offenders recognition that they have conquered us with fear and intimidation, and yes, their power.

For the Princess Anastasia, power came through marriages, followed by money. One source of power she had not known or understood was the physical power that came from intimidation and punishment. Her armor had been her position, as her social connections had been a thoroughfare that detoured past the ugliness of the commoners' lives, leaving her with many enemies.

As Sonya had learned from Madame Natalia, revolution was coming on swift swords in a matter of weeks. Certain members of the aristocracy aligned with the Bolsheviks physically and financially to ensure safe passage out before the coup d'état. The military leaders placed no political significance on women, so to accept their money was sweet sauce on the unnecessary dessert cake.

Sonya had her own protector. Karl, a member of the revolutionary vanguard, promised her safe passage to Paris where she would stay until he summoned her back when he believed she would be safe. She had her own ideas, however. Little did Karl know that his intention and her reciprocity were not compatible.

Madame Natalia resolved not to return to Russia. Her age, she remarked to Sonya, gave her clarity that where one lives out one's remaining days is irrelevant to the security of home and physical comforts. She stunned Sonya by informing her that the destination she chose was a remote area in the southwestern United States named Arizona. Sonya wondered if it was even civilized there, or would Madame Natalia have to contend with shoot-outs on dirty, unpaved roads? As incredible as it sounded, Madame Natalia would not be dissuaded.